Combatting Cellulite

Violetta Schuba

Combatting Cellulite

Meyer & Meyer Sport

Original title: Aktiv kontra Cellulite
– Aachen: Meyer und Meyer Verlag, 1999
Translated by Jean Wanko

British Library Cataloguing in Publication Data
A catalogue for this book is available from the British Library

Schuba, Violetta:
Combatting Cellulite/ Violetta Schuba.
– Oxford: Meyer & Meyer Sport (UK) Ltd., 2001
ISBN 1-84126-032-0

© 2001 by Meyer & Meyer Sport (UK) Ltd.
Oxford, Aachen, Olten (CH), Vienna, Québec, Lansing/Michigan, Adelaide,
Auckland, Johannesburg, Budapest
Member of the World
Sport Publishers' Association (WSPA)
www.w-s-p-a.org

Cover Photo: Fotostudio Schelhaas, Maintal-Dörnigheim
Photos: Anne Schelhaas, Maintal-Dörnigheim
Illustrations: Gregor Krakowiak, Bad Soden-Salmünster,
Cover design: Walter Neumann, N&N Design-Studio, Aachen
Cover and type exposure: frw, Reiner Wahlen, Aachen
Editorial: Winfried Vonstein
Printed and bound in Germany
by Burgverlag Gastinger GmbH, Stolberg
ISBN 1-84126-032-0
e-mail: verlag@meyer-meyer-sports.com
www.meyer-meyer-sports.com

Contents

Preface

The 1990s are characterized by an increased awareness of one's health. Specialized information, especially with regard to prevention is very much in demand, because minor problems often develop into more serious illnesses. The topic "cellulite" is just such a problem, which is receiving more and more publicity and is no longer purely a female problem. Compared with years gone by, where cellulite was regarded merely as a cosmetic change in one's skin, it is now recognized as an illness in many specialist circles. The reasons for this are mainly to be found in how cellulite occurs.

Time and again the blame is put on lack of movement and wrong diet. When the right amounts of sport activities are used correctly, this can help. This is the authoresses starting point, who shows, using numerable exercise examples based on her many years of experience, how our muscles can be strengthened.

Personal motivation is of paramount importance, because it is mainly due to correct application, regularity and consistency, that problems can be prevented or alleviated. More and more gymnastic and sports clubs belonging to the German Gymnastics Association offer sport which specifically strengthens the muscles in these problem areas. Professional instruction, as well as exercising and training together with like-minded people, not only stimulates motivation, but also the psychological well-being of the participants. However, do not expect immediate success.

This book is intended as a guide for your personal use at home as well as in a club.

Pia Pauly   *Dr. Gudrun Paul*
Section leader   *Project Associate*
Department of General Gymnastics

Introduction

Cellulite is a typically female problem. However, what was originally well thought out by Nature, can often lead to the well-known external appearance of an "orange skin" or "mattress phenomenon". By this we mean little cushions or hollows, which are generally to be found in the thighs, bottom, hips, stomach and upper arms. Larger cells of fat lurk behind these uneven indentations which then press freely against the upper surface of skin due to weakness in the connecting tissues and many other factors.

Women with a pronounced cellulite factor are often considerably affected by it. Apart from all the recently published sucking away of fat, it is important to take careful note of the four principles in treating cellulite: *a balanced diet, sufficient exercise, reduction of stress and cosmetic care of the problem areas.*

A firm bottom, firm thighs, a flat stomach and slim hips are what every woman dreams of. The person who does regular sport or exercises, watches what he/she eats, looks after his/her body and relaxes, is doing a good contribution towards healthy circulation, as well as keeping the skin fit. The problem areas would become less a problem by this.

To give us a better understanding of caring cellulite and of prophylactic measures, the book offers wide-ranging, practical endurance and muscle training alongside easy background information on building up one's skin, how cellulite occurs and what to eat. The programme of exercises, aimed at the problem areas, is suitable for all age groups. Innumerable diagrams illustrate the exercises, which are easy to do.

Regardless of what kind of person you are, there is the right solution for everyone. Even if you are currently dissatisfied with your appearance, you can change your body.

My special thanks go to the SCHMIDT Sports Company, the DEHAG Comany and PHILIPS Company Ltd. for supporting us with materials, and to the German REEBOK Company Ltd. for suitable clothing.

I would also like to convey my warmest thanks to Pia Pauly and Dr. Gudrun Paul of the German Gymnastics Association who enabled the publication of this book.

Thanks also go to my photographer, Anne Schelhaas, for the excellent photos and her kind attention.
Finally, my family deserves the most thanks for all their help and support.

Hanau, July 1998
Violetta Schuba

Part I

GENERAL INFORMATION

1 Cellulite - What Is It?

Examining certain parts of a body carefully, one could be put as fatty, despite of one's having an ideal weight. This means that even slim women suffer from cellulite. "Cellulite" means a disturbance in one's natural metabolism. This "disturbance" affects the lymphatic system and the supply of minerals to the tissues. In the encyclopedia, it is described as the absorption of fat into the connective tissues with slight lymphatic congestion and a little oedena (i. g. wastage) in the connective tissues.

This leads to hollows mainly in the thighs, bottom, stomach, hips and upper arms, which resemble an orange skin on closer observation. It is called the "orange" or "mattress phenomenon". Once it was common to regard cellulite in medical circles as a purely cosmetic change in the skin, but today cellulite is at the centre of innumerable discussions an investigations and is even described as an illness by some authors.

The term "cellulite" was first coined in 1812 by Dr. W. Balfour in France and I regard it as the best choice of word for this skin change. There is a whole range of terms for cellulite e.g. *Panniculosis adiposus* (1904), which means superfluous skin tissue around some fat, or *Lipodystrophy* – disturbed metabolism, *Dermopanniculosis deformans* – distorted formation of skin and tissue, *Status protrusis cutis* - skin bulging forward. The term *"cellulitis"* is equally incorrect, because we are not talking about cell inflammation, but rather a disturbance in the metabolism around the sub-cutaneous tissue.

1.1 A Woman's Body Then and Now

The conception of what is beautiful has changed again and again down the decades. For centuries, chubby thighs transformed by cellulite were regarded as attractive in women of which there are numerous examples from ancient times. From around 3000 B.C., the Egyptians were the first people to use skin cosmetics to keep themselves young and slim. So, being fat was out. Then alternated successive waves of slimness with phases of corpulence again being attrative. The great artists in the periods of the Renaissance and Baroque like Leonardo da Vinci, Rembrandt or the famous Flemish painter, Peter Paul Rubens, drew fat-tummied women with big round faces, cellulite arms and thighs, who were regarded as characters of beauty and well-being.

During the Age of Industrialization in the last century, the narrow waist which could be laced up to 45 cm was introduced, but this was counterbalanced by ample hips. For our grandmothers, who often had to go hungry during the war and post-war years – a time of rationalization – fuller, ample and more plump figures were thought to be beautiful. The remark: "Hey, you're looking good", referred to a well-formed person and hence a "female", well-fed body.

Modern art mainly shows intellectual women who are anorexic. The woman of the 60s tried to be like men in many spheres of her life. Her body showed extremely narrow hips and almost a boy-like bottom. This Unisex trend is still with us especially in the cosmetic and fashion world. (e.g. parfume or jeans for both him and her).

After the super-slim anorexic figure of the 70s, a new trend came towards a strong woman with a firm, muscular and well-defined body. The fitness industry of the 90s had returns of thousands of millions and the term "fitness" could be read daily in every magazine. Advertising campaigns present us teenagers with incredibly long, slim cellulite-free legs, having no problems with their figure and who are able to indulge in all "sins" of the world.

Being slim is talked about in the same sense as beauty and health. By no means however every slim woman has a great charisma and is top fit and healthy! A few other things need to be considered.

Slimness is still seen to be a desirable goal, but what if you are not hungry until half past nine in the evening? Should you always resist the dilicious pizza from the Italian take-away round the corner? No, in my opinion, that's wrong. If you decide on a piece of Black Forest Gateau or a delicious chunk of pizza, then you should have the right to enjoy it.

1.2 Stages of a Woman's Life

Childhood

A baby's arms and legs already appear soft, tender, but also plump. So the first signs of cellulite are visible due to a high concentration of hyaluron acid in a child's skin. Hyaluron acid, an important element of the basic mass of connective tissue can absorb a lot of water and can already lead to an increase of child's fat cells by unhealthy diet. Thus it is important to watch a child's diet carefully because "puppy fat" can lead to undesirable overweight when growing up.

Puberty

The "female shapes" come about as a normal part of a woman's development and the ever-changing hormonal situation. The first major change in the female body occurs during puberty, the most difficult time in a developing human being. Girls now suddenly need a bra for their hitherto flat chests and their first monthly period comes overnight. Then their first spots which young eyes immediately see as the very worst outbreak of acne and which are a hindering nuisance on one's first date! Slowly some girls also become aware of words such as "cellulite" or "jodhpur figure". During puberty, oestrogen is first released from the ovaries thus activating the ability of reproduction. Fat level rises and the production of oestrogen increases one's appetite. Also because of the higher oestrogen level, and a small amount of progesterone, the body starts to retain more fluid. This proess can be enhanced by the ovulation-free cycles which often occur in young girls. Progesterone, on the other hand, counteracts the bloated effect of the oestrogen, and not before the end of puberty the hormonal imbalance has stabilized itself. The increased size of the fat cells and the higher concentration of fluid can increase pressure on the blood vessels and thus cause poor circulation in the tissues.

The anti-baby pill

The pill is usually considered when looking for the safest and most widespread form of contraception for young people. A combination of oestrogen and progesterone however can favour water retention and the accumulation of fatty deposits in the tissues, thus causing cellulite. A further disadvantage of this kind of contraception are so-called "broom twigs" in the legs, which can occur when being older.

Pregnancy

Pregnancy is a wonderful time for a woman, especially when she really wants the child. During the first weeks of pregnancy, the hormone progesterone is released in large quantities to keep the womb muscles quiet and prevent their rejecting the embryo. At the same time, the hormone has a calming effect on the whole organism. So tiredness and sleepiness at unusual time are one of the side-effects of progesterone. Thus we can see one of the positive effects of being pregnant: cellulite recedes as a result of the hormones, i.e. water retention and weight increase are not a permanent feature. At this time in their lives, women can take various precautions to avoid excessive weight increase and water retention. Keeping active and eating healthy do good for both, mother and child.

Premenstrual syndromes (PMS)

Just the same month in month out: whether it be a slight headache or stomach cramps   almost every woman regards these monthly complaints as inevitable. Her chest tightens, her stomach longs for a hot water bottle and her whole body feels as if she had put on weight overnight. She can flare up over nothing in particular showing that her psyche is affected. We are talking about the "premenstrual syndrome" which occurs a few days before menstruation. This is caused by hormone variations during the female cycle, where an imbalance takes place between the hormones oestrogen and progesterone, resulting in a build-up of water in the legs and hip areas, which can subsequently make the cellulite hollows worse. One's weight can increase by as much as two kilos.

The Menopause

In fitness studios, one often meets women of well over 50, whose bodies are fit, who look attractive and who radiate the picture of health. When inquiring for the age, one is often surprised about and asks what makes this possible. These women are at a point in their lives, which they often fear because it leads to a dramatic change in the familiar and professional career. However, everything now depends on what management strategies one has learnt so far in one's life. If you have learnt to enjoy life, then you've now got more time for yourself and can indulge yourself more. Just before the change, the oestrogen levels are high and a cycle can take place without ovulation, indicating that one's hormone supply is imbalanced. During the menopause the hormone supply is stabilising;

water retention clearly recedes as also does cellulite. Cellulite goes but then osteoporosis may come in its place. The hormonal change can cause bone wastage, and this can only be prevented by continuing to do specific gymnastics and keeping to a healthy diet. Sexual relations can be enjoyed to the full without any fear of becoming pregnant. The prerequisite, however, for being happy as you get older is a loving life-partner and intact family life.

The mature skin
Our skin is like a well-worn dress which reflects our whole life i.e. we receive the bill for all that we have done wrong or at least haven't always done right. A visible maturing of the skin starts around the age of 30, to which we can add external influences like sunshine, wind, weather, chemical substances,...etc. which all leave their marks.

A mature skin belongs to mature people. When becoming older, the body is not as well supplied with blood as before. When the circulation deteriorates, the skin is becoming older, because less blood in the skin means less nourishment for its cells. It needs longer to recover from injuries, because the skin cells of older people divide more slowly, causing the skin to become thinner. The fat deposits under the skin also become thinner. As well as fat, the water deposits in the cells diminish. The collagen becomes less elastic and the fat and sweat glands become tired, resulting in the skin's losing its moistness and suppleness. All in all, the skin loses its tension which causes creases to occur. Fast aging is a product of many different factors which affect each other i.e. lack of exercise, faulty diet, illnesses, stressed psyche. Just think of future problems which you could avoid, by changing over now to good eating habits, and physical and mental activity.

1.3 Stages of Cellulite

Cellulite is almost a nightmare for many women. Even in the beautiful, slim models one admires daily in many magazines, "orange skin" can be detected under unfavourable light conditions. It is difficult to give a clear description of the various stages of its development, as the reasons and manifestations of cellulite have still not been adequately researched so far. Cellulite is divided into three stages of development: the slight, moderate and severe form.

1. **Slight cellulite** – clear hollows and furrows occur if you pitch the skin. Slight distortions can be seen during normal standing, sitting or lying down.

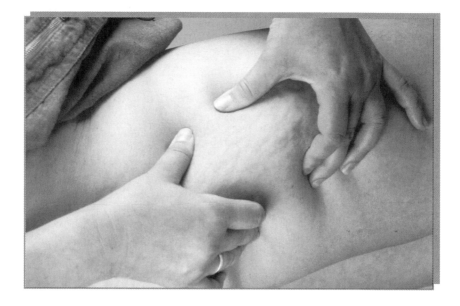

2. **Moderate cellulite** – can be seen in the thighs, hips and bottom when lying down, sitting and standing. Pressure pain in the skin can occur in any of those areas.

3. **Severe cellulite** – when lying down, standing and sitting, deep skin distortions are visible which feel hard and unelastic to the touch. The tissue appears thicker and corny. Unpleasant feelings of tension and heaviness occur in the arms and legs (21)

Specialist doctors refer to this third stage as lipodemia, which is indicated by a symmetrical swelling of the legs, rarely of the arms. Lipodemia can also cause a diffused increase of the subcutaneous fatty tissue with "absorbed" liquid. This is thought to be caused by hormonal influences. Lipodemia usually occurs in late puberty and in 40% of all cases one can find a heriditary tendency.

1.4 Cellulite in Children, Young People and Men

Small hollows and furrows can even occur in the skin of children and young people. If children are overweighted, one can see the cellulite changes best on their tummy. Enlarged fatty cells in the childhood can stay that way and lead to chronic overweight when they are grown up. Men can also suffer from cellulite especially around the waist, whereas women collect their superfluous fat around hips and thighs.

2 Our Skin Under the Microscope

The skin is the largest human organ measuring about 1.7 square metres in size and weighing between 3.5 and 4.5 kilos.

At its thickest point e.g. the back, the soles of one's feet and palms of one's hands, it has between 3 and 5 mm and at its thinnest point, e.g. the eyelids, it has less than 1mm. Through its various layers, the skin fulfills many and various functions:

1. **A protective function** – by the epithel's horniness and by glandular secretions, it protects from mechanical, thermal and chemical damage.

2. **Temperature regulation** – regulation of the body's temperature by vasodilation and vasocontraction, as well as by secreting fluid via the skin's glands.

3. **Water balance** – protection against fluid loss, as well as by secreting fluid and salt via the glands.

4. **Sensory function** – skin sensory organs in the form of pain, pressure, touch and temperature receptors.

5. **Communication** – e.g. blushing, going pale as an expression of vegetative reactions (7).

The human skin-cover consists of the **skin** (cutis) and **subcutis**:

1   Within the skin, one differentiates between an **upper skin** and a **leathery skin**, where each of these layers is composed of various layers of cells.

1a The **epidermis** (upper skin) together with the epithel forms the uppermost layer of the body's surface. In the form of papillary strips it appears a predetermined pattern of lines. The epidermis has three layers, in its lowest layer (basal layer), new cells are constantly being produced (regeneration layer). On the way up to the surface, the cells hornify and produce scales. The melanocytes are found in this layer, which are big cells containing pigment (melanin) and which can be stimulated by increased sunrays to cause the skin to turn brown. They need about two weeks to reach the surface.

1b **The dermis** (leathery skin) mainly consists of a fine network of collagen and fibres, through which blood vessels, sweat glands, sebaceous glands, nerves and hair roots are intertwined. This layer gives the skin its resistance to tearing and the ability of forming. The thicker this network is, the firmer, smoother and healthier the skin appears.

Collagen and elastin fibres are structures which appear in the loose (e.g. dermis connective tissues), elastic (e.g. dermis connective tissues, blood capillary walls) and firm (e.g. ligaments and tendons) connective tissues. They form open-weave nets whose functions comprise: – connecting the organs together, covering parts of muscles, making a guiding framework for branching-off of the blood and lymphatic vessels as well as the nerves.

In the fine blood vessels (capillaries) the most important circulatory function takes place including the exchange of nutrients and cellular metabolic products.

2. **The subcutis** mainly consists of loose connective tissue, that is built up on fatty tissue. This layer enables the skin to move and thus produces energy reserves for the body. The subcutaneous tissue is differently constructed depending on where it is e.g. one talks about "building fat" on the soles of the feet or "depot fat" on the stomach. Its other functions are to protect the internal organs, guard against heat loss, to cushion against pressure and to give the body its shape. Between the dermis and the skin are blood vessels, which stretch out into the cornified layer (7).

Section through the human skin

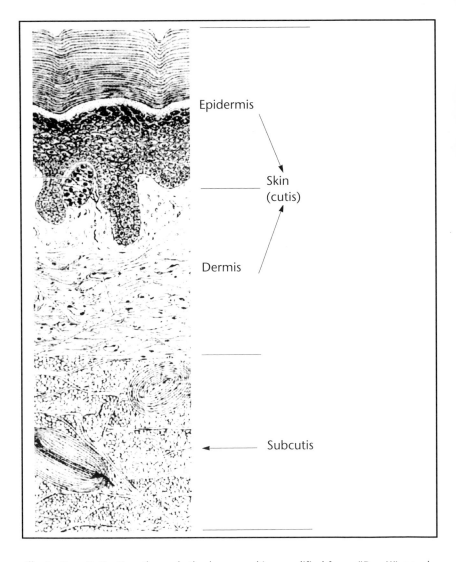

Epidermis

Skin (cutis)

Dermis

Subcutis

Illustration 2: Section through the human skin, modified from "Der Körper des Menschen" dtv, 1995, p.470.

2.1 The Slight Difference Between Male and Female Skin

The different sexes are not only determined by the 23rd chromosome, which with men consists of an X and an Y chromosome, but with women of two X chromosomes. Optically as well as biologically there are many differences as you can see from the following examples:

1. **Brain** – women are more eloquent, have better-connected thought patterns and can put their feelings into words better. However, they have problems with backing into a parking space, listening to loud music and singing to it at the same time. Men master complex activities better.

2. **Hair** – Women lose less hair, as their hair is implanted more firmly, 2 mm deaper than men's hair.

3. **Heart** – if both are untrained, then her endurance capacity is lower; a woman gets out of breath sooner because her heart is smaller although it beats faster.

4. **Liver** – alcohol has a more powerful and long-lasting effect on women, due to the assumption that a woman's liver has less enzymes for getting rid of it. Also, hers is smaller with a lower blood supply.

5. **Metabolism** – women get fat more quickly, because their turn over of energy is less than with men: for the same body weight, they use 700 calories less per day.

6. **Skin** – the structural elements of the skin are the same with men and women, but men have a "thicker skin" than women. Because of its strong epidermis men's skin is better resistant to environmental stresses (e.g. sun, cold). A man's connective tissue is firmer due to less elastin but more smooth muscle fibres. Women get lines and creases earlier because their skin is 0.15 mm thinner and has less fat and sweat glands.

The connective tissue with women is wrapped round little lobes. These lobes or fat cells form upright arches directly connected to the underside of the skin. The tips of the lobes can thus be seen on the surface of the skin as cellulite. However, in men the connective tissue is more strongly anchored in a horizontal position forming a sort of fence-like structure, and the fat cells are settled in little polygons.

Female Skin

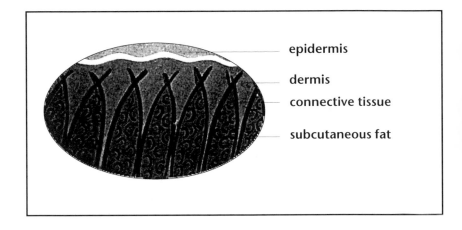

Male Skin

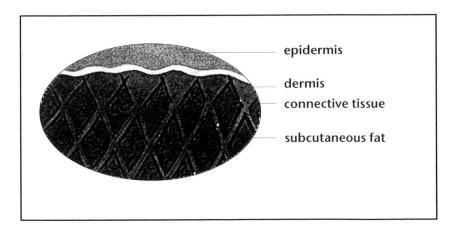

*llustration 3: The slight difference between male and female skin
modified from BURKE, K., 1995, p. 18.*

Cellulite Skin in a Woman

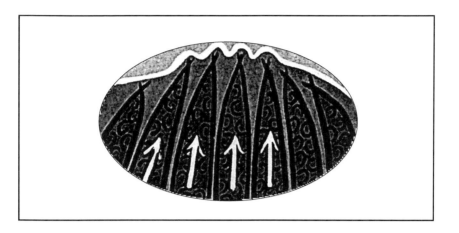

Cellulite Skin in a Man

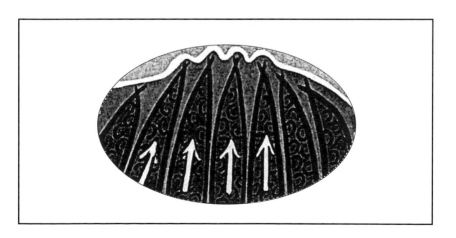

Illustration 4: Cellulite in men and women
modified from BURKE, K., 1995, p. 19.

2.2 Cell Metabolism

Of all chemical compounds in the organism water has the most percentage. The body of an adult human being is made up of about 60% water, which is divided in two different areas: the intra- and extra cellular area.

In the **intra cellular area** (the totality of the volume contained in all the cells) one can find about 2/3 of the body's total fluid (7).

The remaining third is to be found in the **extracellular area** (the totality of the available volume outside of all the cells) and flows round the cells from the outside. Out of these approximately 14 litres of extracellular fluid, about 10.5 litres are to be found in the fine dividing areas (interstitium), which separate the cells from each other, whereas the rest, about 3.5 litres is in the vascular system (arteries, veins and capillaries) (7).

The amount of water in the body remains constant. This is necessary to avoid disturbing the balance of materials dissolved in the body fluid and is a vital prerequisite for the optimum functioning of all the body's cells. Physiological loss of water, like the production of urine, breathing out or sweating during sport, which on average is about 1.5 litres per hour, have to be compensated by drinking. People, who don't fill up their fluid reserves in time are less fit and, at worst, risk damage to their health.

Materials dissolved in the extracellular fluid are known as electrolytes. The largest percentage of salt is cooking salt (NaCl) with a concentration of 9 g per litre. On the other hand inside the cells, (intracellular fluid), potassium is the dominant electrolyte and the concentration of nitrate is about ten times less than outside. The sensitive balance between nitrate and potassium is responsible for keeping intact your inner system. Too much nitrate (salt) in the body has a bad effect on the water supply, because salt binds about seventy times of its own weight of water. Too much nitrate also leads to a lack of potassium, which can cause bloating and a marked deterioration in the orange skin.

2.3 The Blood and Lymphatic System

The heart, motor of the circulatory system, and the capillary system move and conduct the blood.

As a result of the pumping capacity of the heart (a sucking and pushing function), a constant flow of blood is maintained. The blood circulates in a closed system, the capillary system, which consists of elastic tubes and is divided into the following sections:
1. Arteries (main arteries), which conduct the blood away from the heart.
2. Capillaries (tiny vessels), where metabolism takes place.
3. Veins, which conduct the blood back to the heart and
4. Lymphatic vessels, which transport the body fluid and serve to defence.

All the organs of the body receive their nutrients via the blood as well as they are overtaxed with poisonous materials.

The **lymphatic system** runs parallel to the venous circulatory system. It begins "blind" in the area of the capillaries where it takes in the lymphatic fluid and transports it back into the veins' blood via the lymphetic vessels. There are various reasons why fluid (oedemia) can collect in the space between the cells e.g. a rise in blood pressure, a change in the permeability of the capillaries, or also reduced lymphatic drainage caused by narrowing of the lymphatic vessels. When dealing with varicose veins, we are talking about uneven dilation of the veins with constructional changes in the layers of the walls.
This can lead to insufficient closing of the vein valves and a flowing back of venous blood. If there is insufficient lymphatic drainage, then reverse blockage leads to chronic oedemia.

As a result of increased pressure on the tissue, the arterical blood flow is gradually decreased, resulting in circulatory disturbance. The wrong sort of diet (e.g. too much fat and sugar) can cause similar problems. The bloated fat cells operate then like plugs in the tissue. They press on the blood vessels and reduce the circulation, giving rise to bumps and hollows, which can be seen through the skin. When suffering from oedemia, it is helpful to seek therapy from a specialist who will practise manual lymph drainage.

3 Triggering-off Factors

Although various factors have their effects, our lifestyle is usually the main cause of the problem. Consider briefly how you have spent your day and you may recognize yourself again. We eat, although not being hungry, buy ready-prepared meals or prepare them with too much fat, we eat in a hurry and without leaving enough time to digest our food, because the next appointment is schedulded.

Being under stress, we have sudden craving attacks and grab anything we can find to eat, whilst also smoking and drinking too much for social reasons. Our daily work is often done sitting down and what about our leisure time? Well, it would be good if we could learn something about the need to exercise by watching our children.

There is a whole range of hereditay factors however which can have an unfavourable influence on cellulite and of which we have no control. It concerns constitutional types (body structure), the female hormones, and the structure of connective tissue with women. But there are also triggering-off factors within our control e.g. the blood vessel and lymphatic systems, choice of diet and eating habits, our body weight, the balance of muscle to fat, metabolic illnesses, muscular activity and "distress" (i.e. getting rid of stress).

3.1 The Type of Constitution

We cannot do much to alter our body type as it is fixed in our genes (stocky, athletic or asthenic type). Every woman, of course, would like long, slim legs and narrow asthenic hips with a well formed bust, but unfortunaltely these cannot even be conjured up with the strictest diets. If the pelvis is built broadly then not even the best kind of cosmetic surgery can help.

3.2 The Female Connective Tissue

The skin and connective tissue are different with women than with men. The looser connective tissue enables the fatty cells to be pushed outwards from underneath, so that they are visible. If the fatty cells are large, then they will be visible on the surface of the skin in the form of hollows and bumps without any pressure being applied. (see Chapter 2,1).

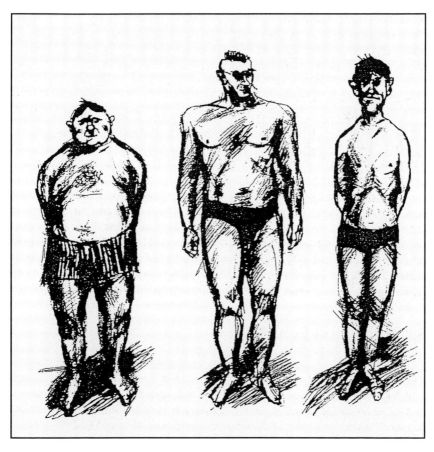

| Stocky type | Athletic type | Asthenic type |

Illustration 5: Somato types: stocky, athletic and asthenic type (by PETER MUSCHALIK, graphic artist from Hindenburg)

3.3 The Hormones

The accumulation of fat and water around the hips and thighs is abetted by the female sex hormones **(oestrogen)**, especially from puberty onwards during pregnancies and during the menopause. Hormonal contraception like the Pill can support this process. On average, a 20-year-old woman has twice as much fatty tissue as a man of the same age. Proportionally, women have about 22 % body fat whereas men have only between 12 and 15 %, which undoubtedly is unfair, but beside others is caused by hormones.

3.4 The Blood and Lymphatic System

The expansion of fatty cells in the lobes of the connecting tissue leads to circulation problems as well as reduced efficiency in the lymphatic system. The reason for this is greater pressure on the vessels, which can result in a "blockage of the body's hydraulic system".

Any fairly long hindrance of the body's circulation can make the cellulite worse. But cellulite is not caused by poor circulation. However, if one has cellulite already, it is unfavourable to the blood and lymphatic circulation.

3.5 Diet and Eating Habits

Too hurried, too fatty, too salty and unbalanced food as well as eating far too much as a result lead to major dietary mistakes and thus to an accumulation of cellulite. Those who have too much water and fat in their tissues will not get rid of cellulite. A diet plan rich in potassium, zine, copper, selerium and silicon can eradicate water in the connecting tissue and, in part, support it to become more tight.

Furthermore it is vital that the body receives an adequate supply of essential nutrients. If a meal is too salty, as a result you have an imbalance in the natrium-potassium pump: if we give our body more natrium (salt) than it needs, water retention occurs and cell activity decreases. Potassium is natrium's natural opponent. Radical dieting may only serve to increase the cellulite problem.

3.5.1 The Free Radicals

A diet rich in fat also helps to support an increase of free radicals. These represent aggressive intermediate products of metabolism and are caused by a small proportion of electrodes which are not finding any contact in the energy combustion process. So they wander about aimlessly, searching for a suitable metabolic partner. So-called anti-oxidants can eliminate these "metabolic terrorists". There are enzymatic anti-oxidants, which need trace elements such as zine, selenium, copper etc. to fulfill their functioning, and non-enzymatic anti-oxidants, which act as water dispensers and neutralize the free radicals thus rendering them harmless. Their most important representatives are vitamin C and E as well as pro-vitamin A.

If fat is burnt up fast (e.g. by radical dieting or extreme forms of sport), far too many free radicals may be released so that vital body structures are under attack. Nicotine, alcohol, too much sun-bathing and increased amounts of ozone can also release too many free radicals.

3.6 One's Body Weight

As cellulite is formed in fatty tissue, we should try to keep this layer as thin as possible. Cellulite is not necessarily synonymous with overweight and yet these two features often are linked. Overweight spoils the body's shape and bulges out extensively the fat cells which are full to bursting. One can reduce the fulness of the fatty cells. However, one's dream of a perfect figure, which we see daily in all the magazines, should not be our ultimate goal, because we cannot alter our own particular bone structure or body type. Crash diets are useless if you wish to lose weight.

3.7 Lack of Movement or Exercise

Muscles which are not in use become floppy. The circulation of blood deteriotes and the muscles do not get enough oxygen. Fatty tissue can best be burnt off with the aid of oxygen, which in practice, means giving it an increased supply of oxygen by doing sport. Especially endurance sport has the most favourable influence. Sitting or standing for long periods of time leads to an accumulation of water in the lower extremities.

3.8 Inherited Factors

The structure of our connective tissue as well as our blood circulation is genetically fixed which means that cellulite can be inherited. However, if a mother has cellulite and thus her daughter also could be susceptible, the daughter could take some precautions. We all "inherit" a certain way of life from our parents, which often remains with us throughout our lives. However, if this is unhealthy we should change it, because these learnt habits encourage orange-skin much sooner than any specific genetic factor. It is all too easy to blame genetic inheritance for our weaknesses.

Scientific investigations throughout the world in both men and women have shown that cellulite occurs in all cultures, although it is found more often in Southern Europe than in the Northern Hemisphere. The reason for this is the habit of diet.

3.9 Stress

Each person needs some essential eustress in order to live and work productively. If distress predominates however, general feelings of frustation, alienation and helplessness get worse, resulting in an increase of innumerable detrimental effects like chronic tiredness, weakend immune system, high blood pressure and burning-out of various body systems.

Distress also has a negative effect on the hormonal system e.g. the adrenal gland, which regulates our water supply and can, if not being careful, encourage water retention. Many people under stress have attacks of sudden craving, which means a supply of too many calories and thus open the door to cellulite. We must realize that WE are the reason of the problem and it does not come by itself.

The body doesn't need much, but it does need quality. The problem is that we have too much of all good things, causing us to disturb our sensitive metabolic mechanism by behaving in a chaotic way. For example, it is not until we get stomach ache from eating too much that we finally realize that we have had too much of the good things.

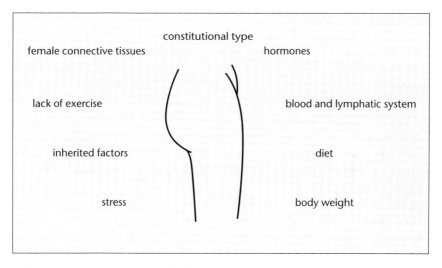

Diagram 6: Factors causing cellulite

4 Body Structure

It is "in" to be slim. Body weight has acquired an almost magical sense in our fitness-orientated society. So, only one thing counts: slim, slim, slim and such an elongated face, longer and longer like an abstract painting. Models are our example, although only 1.3 % of women fit into this body size, and in addition a whole army of stylists and make-up artists lurk in the background of a top model. The scales can either tip in favour of joy, frustation or even depression.

People often put a lot of effort into trying to get their ideal weight. But what is one's ideal weight at a certain age and certain height? And what is the optimum balance of fat to muscles? It is not easy to answer these questions, as there are various theories and opinions on the subject.

4.1 Methods of Determining One's Body Structure

Depending on how we look at it, there are various parameters which determine our body structure. These may be, for example, chemical, metabolic or anatomical components. Water and protein are found mainly in muscles, whereas fat and minerals appear mainly in bones. The simplest and commonest method of describing the human structure is the Double-Component-Method, which distinguishes between the amount of fat and the amount of body (e.g. muscles, heart and circulatory system).

The fatty tissues and the muscles are the most variable components of the body's structure, as, during endurance or strengthening training, the proportion of muscles can be increased whilst the proportion of fat decreases. One's body weight can remain the same, however. Many fitness trainers see this in their participants, who are often frustated by their steady weight.

There are many methods available for measuring the body structure. *Computer-tomography, the X-Ray methods, Weighing under water, infrared measurement, the electrical-conduction method or measuring the thickness of skinfolds with a caliper,* by all of which the relation between muscle mass and subcutaneous fat is determined. The caliper method, has proved to be the best and most-often-used both from a time, financial and equipment point of view. It is also easy to do.

4.2 Measuring Subcutaneous Fat with a Caliper

A very easy long-established practice in English-speaking countries for determining amounts of body fat is by **measuring skinfold-thickness** by using a skinfold **caliper**. This is an exact and very handy instrument for determining the amounts of fat. The subcutaneous fat surrounded by skin is measured in millimeters, and there are various ways of doing this, whereby ten, five, four or even only three points are measured.

A skinfold is pulled up with the fingers together with its subcutaneous fat and its thickness is measured with a caliper. The measurement of the fold's thickness gives us a percentage of how much fat there is in the body and also whether this is low, ideal, average or obese.

There are certain established norms for the ideal proportion of body fat, whereby the following data may be regarded as ideal from a health point of view.

		Women	Men
Age	17-29	25%	15%
	30-39	27.5%	17.5%
	40-49	30%	20%
	over 50	30%	20%

The skin folds together with their subcutaneous fat are pulled up with the fingers at certain points of the body and then measured with the caliper. For the 3-point-method these are the triceps, hip-bone suprailiac and abdomen-skinfold.

Only the total of the three skinfolds can give the approximate amount of subcutaneous fat. You cannot measure yourself at these points. The measuring person takes the caliper in his/her hand and grasps the skinfold to be measured about 1 cm above the measuring point with the thumb and forefinger of the other hand. The caliper is set at a right angle to the appropriate skinfold and the measurement is carried out. We recommend doing each measurement three times and recording the mean value for further calculations.

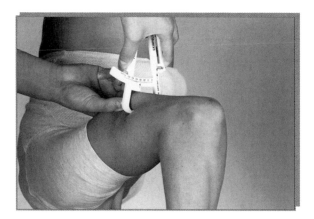

*Diagram 7:
Skinfold of Triceps*

*Diagram 8:
Skinfold of iliac crest*

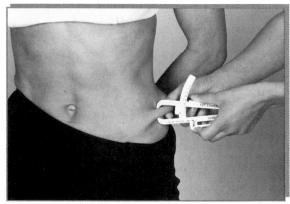

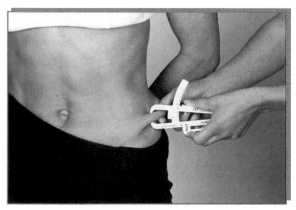

*Diagram 9:
Skinfold of abdomen*

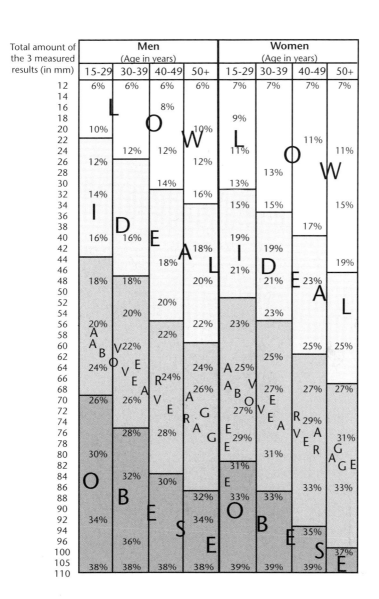

Table 1: Evaluation of the combination of three skin folds.
(Total of the three results)
From: Hautfaltenmesser. Benutzerhandbuch, DEHAG Frechen, p. 20.

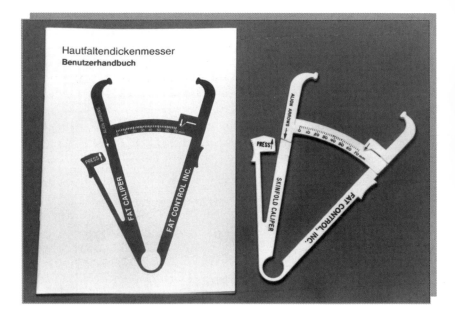

Diagram 10: User's Handbook and Skinfold caliper
Contact: DEHAG Handelsagentur & Verlag, Hermann-Seger-Straße 18-20, 50226 Frechen

5 Body Weight

Our body weight is genetically pre-determined (type of body structure), and also depends on the calorie intake and output to which beside others belong the basic "turnover" or physical exercise. The scales only show the body weight, which just is not specific enough. Scientists have tried to establish some simple ways of evaluating results. The following procedures are the most common, which enable you to find out and evaluate your body weight.

5.1 Normal, Ideal and Well-being Weight

1. Normal weight according to BROCA

$$\text{Height (cm) - 100 = normal weight (kg)}$$

This formula is criticized by dieticians, because there is no differentiation between men and women.

2. Ideal weigth according to a modified BROCA-Index.

$$\text{Women: Height (cm) - 100 - 15\% = ideal weight (kg)}$$
$$\text{Men: Height (cm) - 100 - 10\% = ideal weight (kg)}$$

These strict guidelines are not everyone's "ideal". However, there is a positive relation between a relatively low body weight and innumerable health-promoting effects e.g. advanced life expectancy.

3. Body-mass-Index (BMI)

$$\frac{\text{Body weight = BMI}}{(\text{Height (m)})^2}$$

The standard values:

below 17.9 = underweight

18 - 24.9 = normal weight

25 - 29.9 = overweight (obesity level I)

30 - 39.9 = obesity level II

above 40 = extreme obesity level III

The value for normal weight is a recommendation that does not take sex, age ore one's training condition into consideration.

4. **Well-being weight** means the weight one feels *subjectively* comfortable. This is a body weight, which finds its own level without any special regulations. However, this weight is a serious recommendation, because many biological processes run in their own natural and, above all, individual way. The constraints of modern society and an oversupply can disturb the natural needs of mankind for a long time.

5.2 Under- and Overweight

Around 1% of the population of the Federal Republic of Germany are extremely obese, 16% obese and 40% of the population can be regarded as being overweighted. Due to its frequent existence, obesity (i.e. an abnormal increase in body fat) represents one of Germany's fundamental health problems. It does not only threaten innumerable organic functions, but also leads to serious psycho-social problems. As reasons various genetic, metabolic, cultural, economic and psychological factors are supposed, which overall lead to an imbalance between calorie intake and output. Obesity often starts earlier with men than with women, but when age increases, women are more susceptible to obesity than their male counterparts.

Adiposity can set off and increase many disorders in one's health. Obese people suffer from shortage of breath, get tired faster and have problems with their joints. The conditons are favourable for cardio-vascular risk factors like hypertonia, Type II diabetes, coronary heart attacks and strokes.

Depending on the extent and duration of the overweight these side effects lead to a shortened lifespan. Not only the extent of obesity, but also the distribution of fatty deposits determine the amount of health risk. Men and women with **abdominal** fat distribution have a particular risk for cardio-vascular complications, whereas a **gluteal-femoral** (hip-emphasizing) fat distribution leads to considerably less complications. The reason for this phenomenon is that **visceral** (affecting one's innards) fat cells are more metabolic actively than the subcutaneous ones, which can be found beneath the skin. Enlarged visceral fatty deposits favour the development of the above-mentioned disorders (12) due to an increasing release of fatty acids. The Nurses' Health Study has shown clearly that a 10 kg increase in an adult's weight is not without any risk.

As a result of their situation, many overweight people are often suffering from depression and disorder of self-esteem. Particularly the social disadvantages are a great strain. It has been proved that overweight people have poorer career prospects and a lower income. That is because lack of motivation and other negative characteristics often are implied to overweight. At the end of 1994 a team of Dr. Jeffrey FRIEDMAN from Rockefeller-University succeeded in identifying the **ob-gene** which has a share for obesity. The chromosome number 7 is the information carrier of the individual fat distribution pattern and the place of this gene. The ob-gene (obesity = state of being fat; adiposity) controls and adjusts feelings of being hungry and be filling. It stimulates the fat cells to produce the hormone **leptin** which consists almost entirely of adipocytes and controls the food intake as well as one's energy consumption. The more fat is available, the more leptin is syntheticized. If the production of this hormone is low, the body weight may increase. However, many overweight people do not lack leptin, but have even too much of this hormone in their blood. Possibly a defective hormone receptor, i.e. the ob-gene was the reason that the transmitted messages could not be received. Those people already suffer from adiposity in their childhood, as well as from a high insulin level, which is a result of it and causes feelings of permanent hunger. They are seldom filling because there is something wrong with their regulatory system. Such people need permanent medical treatment. On the other hand the majority of obese people have their fatty rinds by eating too much and therefore they can lose their superfluous pounds again (33, 34, 35).

In surgical therapy of extremely overweight patients, mainly two methods are used: **Mason's vertical gastro-plastic surgery or gastro-plastic surgery with an adjustable stomach band** made of silicone. Surgical therapy is an effective method with a 60-70% success rate. After vertical plastic surgery, patients lose an average of 40 kilos of their body weight in the first 24 months. However, only extremely overweight patients should be operated. The aim of obesity therapy must be to choose patients more carefully for the various kinds of therapies, in order to avoid failure. This involves: dietary measures, behaviour- and psycho-therapy, therapeutic exercises, medicinal therapy and only as a last resort, surgical therapy (17).

The changeover from fanatical dietary, which affects many people today, to a real eating disorder is smooth-running. The critical factor is when you increasingly only think of your weight when eating. You keep on getting on the scales, calculate the calories and feel dreadfully guilty when you have only a piece of cake. Emotionally you feel worse and worse and you withdraw into your shell. Many people secretly take lots of laxatives or are vomitting intentionally.

Anorexia and **Bulimia** are real illnesses, seldom caused by purely physical disease but rather having severe emotional problems as their starting point. Sensitive types of people, who always seek to please others, and who were required a lot of discipline and perfection from an early age on, are particularly endangered. Young, attractive women often find no other outlet for their feelings of helplessness, fear or anger; so they try to overcome an emotional problem at a level of body and food. Especially young people, particularly during puberty, who have little genuine self-esteem, orientate themselves too much outwardly. They like to identify themselves with what is "in" and what other people think and say about them. They are also far too self-critical. Physical damages such as poor circulation, a dry and scaly skin, osteoporosis, renal disorders, as well as renal failure and cardiac arrest can all result from being underweight. If someone has an eating disorder, usually the whole family and environment is affected. Our society is very much success-orientated. Only the slim and super thin persons, who are put on the same level as vitality, beauty, success and self-discipline, are regarded as successful. What is lacking today is a human-being one can lean on at any time and have a good cry, and where one does not have to be perfect!

PART II

ANTI-CELLULITE TRAINING - THEORY

Anti-cellulite training really means taking some active precautions to avoid it. The affected person must take the initiative and study carefully the background to understand it. A complex procedure is necessary to get rid of orange skin and thus act against cellulite: doing endurance sport and some specific muscle strengthening as well as changing your diet and combatting stress. An additional measure is skin care where particulary massage-effects are an important thing. **However, only by working emotional from inside success can be achieved.** Only external measures by themselves will give rise to nothing.

6 Sport

Doing some kind of endurance-orientated sport and specific strength training are one way of actively reducing cellulite.

Endurance sports are the best fat killers and they bring about a permanent optimum body weight and body structure. The longer and more intensively one trains the greater the burning up of calories, and the more muscle groups are dynamically used. Specific strengthening exercises can also tighten and shape the muscles as well as having a positive influence on one's metabolism. The more muscle mass a person has, the more "furnace" he can set in motion for fat metabolism.

It is also important to take care of one's psyche. If the kind of sport moderately done, generates enough sweat, amounts of endomorphine are released producing a good mood, contentment and a euphoric condition. One starts to crave for this kind of home-made good mood, which is one of the least dangerous forms of dependence. Intensive physical exercise lays the basic foundation for health and longevity, influences one's normal weight and ensures an attractive body.

6.1 Endurance

The endurance capacity is dependent on the basic conditional motoric abilities of strength, speed, agility and co-ordination. Depending on the energy release, the endurance capacity can be divided into anaerobic and aerobic. **Anaerobic** means that energy is generated **without oxygen** whereas oxygen is vital in generating aerobic energy. During endurance training, there is always a mixed metabolism of aerobic and anaerobic energy release. During the generation of anaerobic energy, which is uneconomical, high-energy carbohydrates are burnt. **Lactate** (lactic acid) is produced as wastage. If the body is "overacidified", the physical activity must be stopped. During aerobic training, that works by oxygen, carbohydrates and fats are burnt. It is obvious that endurance training has many positive effects on the whole organism.

6.1.1 Positive Effects

Endurance training indisputably is the most important factor in preventive measures as well as in rehabilitation. It improves one's general physical capacity and general well-being. To have positive effects regular training, e.g. two to three times per week is a prerequisite.

Positive effects of endurance training

Heart:	increase of the maximum stroke volume and of the cardiac output, reduced resting pulse-rate, increased maximum oxygen intake, economizing of the heart-work.
Breathing/Lungs:	increase in the vespiratory-volume, improved breathing economy.
Blood/blood vessels system:	improved oxygen supply to the muscles, prevention of arteriosclerosis, reduction of blood-flat, reduced risk of getting thrombosis.
Muscles:	improvement of circulation, oxygen intake and oxygen storage.
Immune system:	strenghtening of the immune system, prevention of tumour disorders.

Risk factors:	prevention of cardio-vascular diseases.
Psyche:	reduction of stress, improvement of one's self-esteem and well-being.
Regeneration:	improved regeneration ability.
Body forming:	reduction of body weight, changes in one's metabolism which counteract the storage of fat, lack of appetite after training, longer "food-free" periods as a result of sport.

6.1.2 Duration and Intensity

The duration as well as the intensity of endurance training depends on the established aim of the trainee. The following goals could be aimed at:

- rehabilitation
- prevention
- reduction of stress
- maintaining or improving fitness
- weight reduction, body shaping
- social contacts

Depending on one's established aim a decision is made to a particular kind of sport, duration and intensity. Endurance training is the best way of reducing body fat, but a particular emphasis is put on the duration of exercise. For this it is better to have a **permanent load over a longer period of time (at least 30 minutes) with less intensity** than a short load duration at a higher intensity. Over 80% of leisure sportsmen train too intensively. Especially during anaerobic training, the balance between carbohydrate break down and fat burning is unfavourable.

During the first half of an hour, it is mainly carbohydrates which are burnt off, as in a metabolic process they can be transformed into energy faster than fat. Only when the load duration is longer the body is using its fatty deposits – this leads to an increased break down of fatty acids and finally to "adipocyte melting".

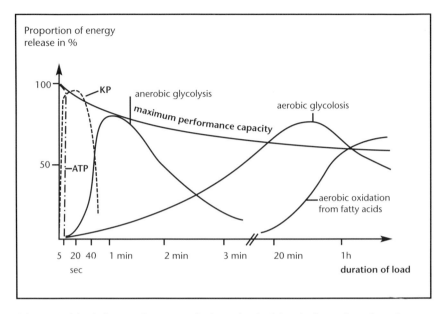

Diagram 11: Release of energy during physical load of varying duration, as well as the maximum performance capacity (from PAUL, G. etc. 1996, p. 41)

In practice, one should have an endurance work of at **least 45 minutes and at most 90 minutes (otherwise overloading of the joint system),** during which the whole body moves (at least a sixth of the skeletal muscles).

The **control of intensity** in endurance training can be raised as follows:
• increased speed of movement
• hilly territory
• wider arm and leg movements
• use of extra apparatus like latex bands or small dumb-bells during interval training.

During exercises to music (aerobics) by:
• increased music tempo
• high-impact steps (e.g. hopping, jogging)
• raising and lowering the body's centre of gravity (e.g. jumping jack)

There are various ways of training one's endurance capacity and any of the following **methods** may be used:

- **The continuous endurance method** – a long-lasting load of at least 30 minutes, without a rest in the training unit, with a heart rate (HR) between 70% and 80% of the maximum HR.

- **The alternating endurance method** – defined sections of a course and periods of time at varying speeds. E.g. 15 mins at 75% HRmax., 10 mins at 85% HRmax. within a 45-minute total extent of loading.

- **The extensive interval method** – systematic alternation of load and recovery phases within a training unit. E.g. 3-6 minutes at 85% - 90% HRmax. and a 2-5 minutes rest (walking/trotting) or until a recovery heart rate of 120/minute is reached.

Interval training is supposed to have a better effect on fat burning than with constant endurance load. The intervals can be set up in different ways. One interval variation: 4-6 minutes endurance training (aerobic) and 2-3 minutes strength training (with small weights/physio bands), the ratio is 2:1.

In the fitness area, the above mentioned methods are used. Various small pieces of apparatus (dumb-bells, bands,...) can be implemented to vary the training programmes and by means of which the intensity of training can be raised. People who are flexible in training hours, should it put of to the mornings.

Results of a study at Kansas University show that in the mornings 2/3 of the calories are burnt off the fat cells, whereas in the afternoons and evenings it is only the half of. The reason is that one trains without a full stomach in the mornings so that there is less carbohydrate available for the energy release.

6.1.3 Heart Frequency Control

An optimum load intensity is necessary in order to avoid overloading, as well as to ensure positive signs of adaptation within the organism. In endurance sports the lactate levels in the blood are the parameters trainers use to plan the training. From a sports medicine point of view, blood lactate levels up to about 4 mmol/l are the most favourable to develop endurance capacity.

A simpler parameter to control the load intensity is to measure one's heart or pulse rate. The heart rate is measured close to the heart, whereas the pulse rate is checked either on the thumb side of the wrist, on one's temple or at the carotid artery. The simplest apparatus is a heart rate monitor which consists of a transmitter in a chest strap and a receiver with display screen. Being able to set the lower and upper limit of training makes it easier to find the right intensity.

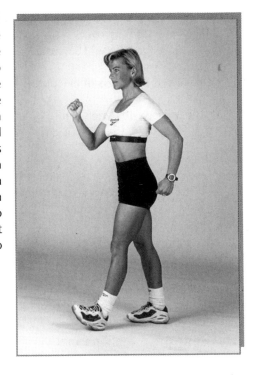

Diagram 12:
Heart rate monitor by "Polar"

There are four heart rate (HR) parameters which are important for realisation of the training and to control the intensity of it.

1. **Resting-HR** – measured straight after your night's sleep still lying down. The resting pulse is best measured for one minute in the mornings (still lying in bed).
   The resting heart rate (recovery area) is about 70-80 beats per minute for untrained people, whereas with trained people it is about 40 beats per minute. Cyclists and triathletes at the peak of their capacity have rates as low as 26-30 beats per minute.

2. **Training-HR** – heart rate measured during load, it depends on the type of sport and can be calculated from the maximum HR. A leisure sportsman trains his basic endurance capacity in a HR area ranging from 60-80% of his maximum heart rate.

3. **Maximum HR** – 220 minus one's age in years (this is only a rough orientation).

4. Recovery HR – the better the endurance capacity, the faster one's cardiovascular system recovers from the load. After about 3 minutes, the heart rate should be below 110 beats per minute.

There are various **methods of calculating the training HR.**

1. Formula in line with one's age:
For untrained people, the following age-related formula applies:

180 – age = training pulse rate

This is the simplest way of calculating the training pulse rate.

2. Standard formula:
The most popular method is the so-called standard formula:

220 – age in years = maximum heart rate

The recommended training should be within 60-80% of the maximum heart rate.

Example of a 33-year-old-person:
220 – 33 = 183 beats/minute as maximum HR
60% = 110 beats/minute
80% = 146 beats/minute
The best training heart rate is between 110 and 146 beats per minute.

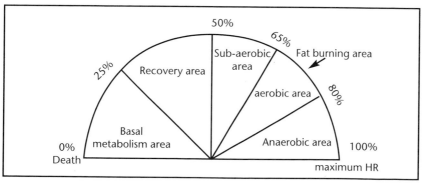

Diagram 13: Training areas related to one's heart rate; modified by: BAILEY, C., 1996, p. 79

3. KARVONEN formula

When using the KARVONEN formula, the calculation is dependent on the resting pulse rate:

$$\textbf{(220 – age – resting pulse) x \% of max. HR = Q}$$
$$\textbf{Q + resting pulse = training heart rate)}$$

Example for a 33-year-old person:
   (220 - 33 - 60) = 127
According to KARAVONEN, the optimum type of training is between 50% and 85% of these calculated data (127) plus the resting pulse rate.

$$\textbf{(127 x 0.5) + 60 = 124}$$
$$\textbf{(127 x 0.85) + 60 = 168 beats/minute}$$

The training heart rate is between 124 and 168 beats/min.

4. Recommendation for training by LAGERSTRØM

For an exact calculation individual variations must be taken into consideration and this is just what LAGERSTRØM does. In addition to the age, the resting pulse rate and the training status as well as the particular type of sport is considered. The following figures are for aerobic training (30):

Endurance sports	Untrained	Moderately Trained	Endurance Trained	Performance Trained
Running Resting pulse + (220 – 3/4 of one's age – resting pulse) x	0.6*	0.65*	0.7*	0.75*
Biking Resting pulse + (220 – age – resting pulse) x	0.6*	0.65*	0.7*	0.75*
Swimming Resting pulse + (220 - age – resting pulse) x	0.6*	0.65*	0.7*	0.75*

* = Factor

Table 2: LAGERSTRØM's recommended training pulse from "Schlank für immer", Fit for Fun 10/97, p. 24

If the emphasis is on burning off fat, the given data can be reduced by 5-10 pulse beats, especially for beginners.

Here is an example for a 40-years-old runner, who is endurance-trained:
$60 + (220 - 30 - 60) \times 0.7 = 60 + (130 \times 0.7) = 60 + 91 = 151$ beats/minute (Training pulse rate)

There is a whole range of factors, which can influence one's pulse rate (heart beats/minute) e.g. age, training status, climate, illnesses, medicines, form of the day, type of sport, terrain. The simplest motto for endurance sport is "running without snorting" or "cycling without getting out of breath", which means gauging the amount of load so that it is possible to hold a coherent conversation with another training partner (speech test).

The following table indicates heart rates for training which are age-related:

Age	Heart Rate - preferred area 60-75% of max. pulse	Maximum Heart Rate max. Pulse 100%
20	120-150	200
25	117-146	195
30	114-142	190
35	111-138	185
40	108-135	180
45	105-131	175
50	102-127	170
55	99-123	165
60	96-120	160
65	93-116	155
70	90-113	150

Table 3: Age-related training ranges

A study has shown that about 80% of all leisure joggers train in the peak of performance range.

Remember: **Sport in itself is not healthy, but only as healthy as you make it.**

6.1.4 Endurance Sports

During cardiac training, one can differentiate between **Outdoor and Indoor Sports**. There is a whole range of endurance apparatus in fitness studios, which are not only intended for warming up, but also can be used as great fat killers. An indoor programme has the following advantages: top-grade apparatus make the training safe and efficient, experienced trainers set up individual programmes and keep an eye on the course of training, varied training can be done on the different kinds of apparatus, motivation is high because the cardiac equipment gives you immediate results (pulse, calorie combustion). One can use the following cardiac equipment: running band, stepper, climber, rowing apparatus, ski trainer, bike (spinning).

The most popular indoor endurance sport is different styles of aerobics.
    Outdoor sports include: inline-skating, cycling, jogging, walking, swimming (aqua-training), hiking, long-distance running, canoeing.

6.1.5 Energy Used During Endurance Sport

The longer and more intensively one trains, the higher the use of calories is up. Here are a few examples of how you can use up energy:

Lying down	4.2 KJ/kg/hour
Standing	6.4
Walking (6 km/hour)	15.5
Cycling (20 km/hour)	32.3
Running (12 km/hour)	45.2

Example:
Jogging, a person of 70 kg runs for 30 minutes at a speed of 10 km/hour.
1. Calculated oxygen uptake (VO_2) during jogging:
   VO_2 (in ml/min/kg) = running speed (km/h) x 3.656 - 3.99

2. VO_2 (in ml/min/kg) = 10 (km/h) x 3.656 - 3.99 = 32.57
   Oxygen uptake is 32.57 ml per minute per kg of body weight.

3. Oxygen uptake 32.57 x 70 kg = 2280 ml/min
   Oxygen uptake data - 2.280 ml/min

4. As 1 kcal correspondents to an oxygen throughput of 200 ml, there is an energy consumption per minute of about 11.4 kcal (2280 : 200 = 11.4 kcal)

5. 30 mins. x 11.4 = 324 kcal

Result:
The jogger uses up 324 calories in 30 mins. at a speed of 10 km/hour (5, Volume 2, p. 80).

In active people, the fat falls by the wayside. The energy used does not depend on the load duration, but on one's body weight. You can read off the approximate calorific consumption per time unit from the data given below. The printed data are averaged over 60 minutes.

Activities	Body Weight	
	50 kg	70 kg
Aerobics	312	441
Window Cleaning	177	248
Football	396	554
Digging the garden	378	529
Inline-Skating	360	504
Jogging (12 km/hr)	624	874
Cleaning	186	260
Cycling (15 km/hr)	300	420
Swimming (breast stroke)	486	681
Dancing (Twist)	312	436
Tennis	327	458
Volleyball	125	210
Hiking (18 kilos of huggage)	300	420

Table 4: Calorific consumption during various activities (60 mins.)

We recommend using up about 2,000 calories per week in sporting activities.

6.1.6 Suggestions for Endurance Training

- Endurance training is possible at any age, but from the age of 35 on we recommend examination by a sports doctor before you start.
- You will only achieve success if you train regularly.
- Big gaps in training can quickly lead to a drop in performance capacity.
- Choose a type of endurance training, which you enjoy.
- Begin slowly and increase gradually, so that you are working for between 30 and 60 minutes.
- If you have any kind of flu-related illness with a temperature, you should avoid all activity.
- Ensure that your last meal was about 2 hours before training.
- If smog or ozone is at a critical level, avoid endurance training or put it of to the early morning or late evening and then at best only in an indoor area.
- Do some relaxed cooling down at the end of each training session, so that your body can regenerate more quickly. Both from a training and sport medicine point of view, there is no sense in putting on a final spurt, because large amounts of lactate are produced, which have a negative effect on your regeneration (5).

6.2 Muscle Strength Training

Endurance training combined with strength training can have a positive effect on fat reduction. The metabolic post-loading effect after endurance training can last for some time and so the adipocytes go on "melting". Specific exercises for problem areas is the second sporting precaution which can strengthen the muscles as well as tightening and remodelling them.

Strength belongs to the five basic motoric functions alongside endurance, flexibility, co-ordination and speed. In the area of basic abilities, one's strength endurance capacity occupies a special place. The advantages of strength training properly carried out are many and various. However, the effects depend on how the exercise is carried out, choice of exercise, amount, method and regularity.

After the age of 30, one's strength potential recedes if it is not adequately stimulated. Many people sit around voluntary "all their lives", if they spend eight hours working at a desk and spend their leisure time being inactive. So, in order to preserve and improve one's strength potential and general load tolerance of one's posture and mobility structure, some specific strength training is indeed necessary.

6.2.1 The Positive Effects of Strength Training

Here are a few advantages of regular strength training:

Prevention
- Precautions taken against weakness in posture, back trouble, osteoporosis, arthritic changes, muscular dysbalance.
- Maintaining and improving one's general capacity and mobility structure.
- Stabilizing the passive mobility structure – increasing the fitness and load tolerance of tendons, ligaments and bones.
- Compensating receding strength as one gets older.

Rehabilitation
- Improvement of the healing process after injuries e.g. slipped discs, torn ligaments, broken bones...
- Reducing the pain with chronic ailments like back ache or knee problems.
- Fast regeneration of performance capacity after lengthy immobile periods caused by injury.

Enhanced performance
- Optimum strength ability and increase in strength is a prerequisite of all kinds of sport.
- When muscular dysbalance has been caused by a particular kind of sport, strength training can compensate for muscles otherwise not specially trained.

Getting the body into shape
- Building up muscle bulk.
- Tightening the tissues and giving the muscles a good profile.
- Reduction of the amount of fat.
- Losing weight (dependent on type of training).
- Increasing weight if underweight.

Psyche
- Development of body awareness and improvement of body sensitive.
- Improving one's self-image.

6.2.2 Types of Strength

The strengthening exercises in sport are for preservation and improvement of the following strength abilities :

- **Strength endurance**
- **Fast strength**
- **Maximum strength.**

The aim of strengthening, in prevention as well as during therapy, is aimed at training the muscles for improving their maximum strength and maintaining their strength. There is little point in training fast strength when one is much older. The greatest strength that the nerve and muscle system is capable of during voluntary contraction is known as **maximum strength**. **Strength endurance** is the ability to maintain tests of strength over a specific period of time. **Fast strength** is the ability to produce the strongest burst of energy within a given time, comprising the following components of starting, explosive and maximum strength.

Muscle-building training (**Hypertrophy training**) of moderate intensity (about 60-75 % of one's maximum strength potential) encourages mainly formation of the bones and muscles if done with moderate to fairly difficult loads. By this, on the one hand, enough powerful stimuli are given to achieve a desired adaption effect, on the other hand, one more or less avoids the danger of overloading if carried out correctly. Muscle-building training can be done with additional apparatus (e.g. physio bands, physiotapes, physio tube rings, physio tube toners, physio power tubes, spiders, weight cuffs, heavy hands etc.) both with and without a partner or at appropriate strength training machines in a fitness studio. If fitness apparatus is used, then the effect of training is enhanced. At the centre of all strengthening exercises should be the specific working at one particular muscle group, which presupposes certain knowledge of how muscles work, as well as understanding the most important weaker groups of muscles.

Groups of muscles which are most prone to **weakness**:
- Anterior neck muscles
- Shoulder blade muscles (Rhomboids, seratus anterior)
- Lumbar extensor muscle in the area of the pectoral vertebrae (erector spinae)

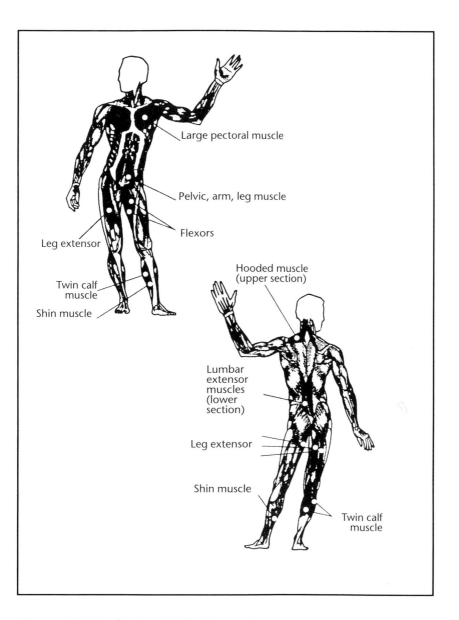

Diagram 14: Muscle groups inclined to weakness.
From PAUL, G./SCHUBA, V., 1997, p. 48

- Seat muscles (glutaels)
- Abdominal muscles (rectus abdominis, obliqui)
- Knee joint extensor muscles (vastus medialis, intermedius, lateralis)
- Anterior shin muscles (tibialis anterior)
- Foot muscles

One of the effects of strength training is to shorten the muscle fibres. If the muscles are not stretched enough after the training session, muscular deficiency or dysbalance can occur, which can cause serious damage to the main joints. The process of degeneration takes place slowly and the painful ailments are often a sign of irreparable damage (see chapter 6.3).

6.2.3 Working Forms of Strength Training

There are two main ways of working in strength training: **static** and **dynamic**, which both have their advantages and disadvantages, but they should be mixed in practice. The dynamic form should have precedence being specifically suited to everyday activity.

Characteristics of static (isometric) strength training:

- The muscle group or the muscle is tensed as much as possible without its joint or origin being approached i.e. without moving the corresponding limbs.

- By isometric tensing, it is possible for a person to produce maximum strength results.

- With this method, the muscle is stimulated by the nerve system to activate all the available muscle fibres, in order to overcome the apparent hindrance.

- Similarly, we recommend isometric exercises in the starting phase of strength training, so that evasive movements do not occur as quickly.

- Tensing exercises also have their **disadvantages**: danger of forced breathing, reduced blood circulation in the muscles, rise in blood pressure, if only this sort of exercise is done, the ability of the muscles to react is reduced and the strength training is angular specific.

Characteristics of dynamic (isotonic) strength training

- In dynamic strength training, we differentiate again between **dynamic-concentric** strength training (overcoming the force of gravity) and **dynamic-excentric** strength training (giving, into the force of gravity).

- Dynamic strength endurance training has a positive effect on the elasticity of the muscles, tendons and ligaments.

- In addition, dynamic strength training promotes the neuro-muscular interplay (co-ordination of muscles and nerves) and thus helps to cope with the demands of all our daily movements.

Pros and cons of both types of training:

STATIC Training	DYNAMIC Training
Pros:	**Pros:**
Easy to do;	Suited to the everyday
Short time involved;	as well as to sport;
Improvement of one's	Improvement of one's
intra-muscular co-ordination	intermuscular co-ordination
(neuro-muscular).	(neuromuscular),
	The muscle power thus
	achieved lasts longer.
Cons:	**Cons:**
Monotonous in the long run;	Difficult to gauge;
No (or only slight) endurance	Frequent evasive movements;
improvement;	
No inter-muscular improvement	Longer build-up phase.
in co-ordination;	
Counter-productive with heart disease;	
Blood supply to the muscles is reduced;	
Angular specific strengthening.	

6.2.4 The Right Amount

How training is set up in the area of strength depends on the aims of the training and the individual requirements of the trainee. All beginners should start with some introductory training with a very low loading intensity, thus avoiding over-straining the body.

Strength endurance and muscle-building training belong to the area of health-orientated fitness training. In strength endurance training we are talking about using a submaximal tension repetition method with lots of repetition. If done correctly, the danger of over-loading is more or less excluded. The level of intensity with this method is between 65 and 30% of the maximum strength (K_{max}) by the trainee; there could be 20-50 repetitions in 3-6 sets with a 3-5 minute rest.

Strength endurance: 20-50 repetitions /3-6 sets/3-5 min. rest

When training for muscle-building (hypertrophic method – method of submaximal tension repetition until one is tired), one trains at an intensity of 60-75% of the K_{max}.

Hypertroph: 8-20 repetitions/3-10 sets/2-5 min. rest

After completing a set, one should feel slightly tired or only a pleasant "burning" in one's muscles.

Performance potential can be increased in both training methods and also some influence in forming one's figure can be achieved.

Fitness-orientated strength training is linked with reducing fat and improving one's figure: the larger the amount of muscles, the more fat burning deposits we have at our disposal.

Careful when dieting: the body does not only get rid of fatty tissue but also of protein (see p. 74).

6.3 Mobility Training

One of the effects of strength training is that it shortens the muscle fibres. Without any **stretching**, their molbility deteriorates. As we get older, the loss of mobility in our spine, our shoulder and hip joints inhibits us more and more in our everyday activities as well as in sport.

The frequent neglect of the basic motoric characteristic – "optimum mobility" – can be seen in fitness centres, where more emphasis is on endurance and strength training. This is despite the fact that mobility training is already several thousand years old.

At the end of each training session, muscle groups which have had a particularly intensive workout should be adequately stretched.

The following groups of muscles are inclined to **shortening**:

- Shoulder and neck muscles (Trapezius downhill section)
- Pectoral muscles (Pectoralis)
- Lumbar extensor (Erector spinae in the hip and neck area)
- Hip bender (Iliopsoas)
- Adductors
- Knee joint extensor (Rectus femoris)
- Posterior thigh muscles (Hamstrings; Ischiocrurales)
- Calf muscles (Gastrocnemius, Soleus)

"**Stretching**", introduced from the U.S.A. and presented in book form by Bob Anderson in 1980, has led us to a complete turnaround in our opinion on all muscle-stretching exercises in each and every kind of sports warming up programme. Bouncing stretching exercises are condemned, and "gentle" slow stretching hailed as the one and only healing method for becoming "flexible".

Innumerable investigations in recent years led to the conclusion that rhythmic-dynamic stretching (intermittently) could also have a positive effect. KRAFT and others (20) discover that intermittent stretching improves the "relaxibility" of the muscle, whereas static stretching makes it worse.

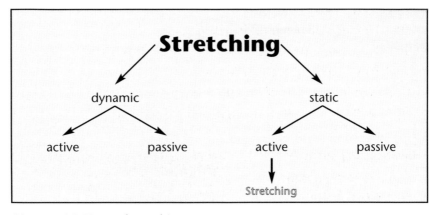

Diagram 15: Types of stretching
dynamic = springing or bouncing
static = stretching position is held
active = the stretching is brought about by contraction of the opposing player
passive = without any muscular effort, with the help of apparatus, or of a partner or one's force of gravity

Stretching is the static, active kind of stretching, also known as "held stretching".

6.3.1 The Effects of Stretching

The morphological characteristics of muscle and connecting tissues, just like the neurophysiological ability to steer or guide are positively influenced by stretching:

- Stretching enhances the load ability of a muscle, so that a greater reach can be reached by the corresponding joint.

- Stretching reduces the resting tension of a muscle, so that the muscle allows a longer reach of the corresponding joint owing to less opposition from the stretching force.

- Stretching lengthens the muscle, so that it allows a longer reach of the corresponding joint because of its increased length.

- Stretching improves the relaxability of the muscle.

- Stretching prevents injuries.
- Stretching gets rid of muscular dysbalance.
- Stretching speeds up the rehabilitation process after injury.
- Stretching speeds up regeneration.
- Stretching improves the body's general sense of wellbeing.
- Stretching improves the sporting performance ability.

6.3.2 Stretching Methods

1. **Static stretching (SS):**
   The muscle is stretched. After 10-30 seconds of keeping the same stretching position, the muscle is slowly relaxed. This procedure may be repeated.

Example: the ischiocrural muscles (back of thigh) are stretched by bending the body forward (keeping the back straight).

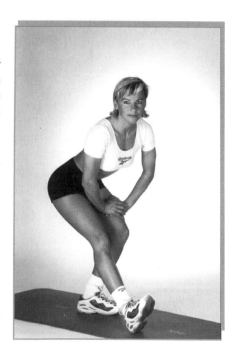

Diagram 16: Stretching the ischiocrural muscles

2. **Contraction-Relaxation-Stretching (CR):**
   At this method, a 10 second absolutely static contraction of the appropriate muscle precedes the stretching process of that same muscle. After 2-3 seconds of continuous relaxation, comes the same stretching as in static stretching.

Example: First tense the ischiocrural muscles for 10 seconds, then relax and proceed as for static stretching.

3. **Antagonistic-Contraction-Stretching (AC): –**
   This stretching begins with static stretching. When the maximum stretching position has been reached, the antagonistic muscle is contracted as far as possible for a duration of about 10-20 seconds. The stretching position is thus lowered. Then gradually relax the stretching position.

Example: Start with static stretching and when the maximum stretching position of the antagonist has been reached, i.e. the front of the thigh (M. quadriceps femoris), then relax. Maintain tension for 10-20 seconds.

The three stretching methods are frequently combined with each other and modified (20, 36).

7 Diet

The second pillar of cellulite prevention is a balanced diet. Our way of life and eating habits are often the root cause of cellulite. So, what does a balanced diet really mean, and what is a particularly effective way of getting rid of water and waste products in tissues in the problem areas? How many calories does the body need per day?

These are just a few of the questions with no easy answers. In recent years, biochemists have ascertained that innumerable healthy products are to be found in fruit and vegetables, which offer help in combatting virtually every disease in all sorts of different combinations. We musn't forget that mankind is naturally equipped first of all to nourish himself from plants and then from meat.

In this chapter we will introduce certain food products, especially rich in substances which combat cellulite.

7.1 Food Products

Central to a healthy and balanced eating plan are fresh, lean and nourishing food products. It is true that carbohydrates, proteins and fats all contain vital ingredients of a balance diet, but one's need for these varies. The German Food Society makes the following recommendations.: **55-60% from carbohydrates, 15-20% from protein and 25-30% as fat.** In addition to this, the body needs enough minerals such as potassium, calcium phosphate, sodium, trace elements like iodine, iron, selenium... and vitamins e.g. vitamin A, the B vitamins, vitamin C, D and E,... .

7.1 1 Carbohydrates, Fats and Proteins

Carbohydrates are the muscle fuel of any sportsman. He gets it from simple sugars like glucose, fruit and household sugar and double combined sugar (milk sugar and malt sugar) which supply energy quickly but only for a short time as well as compound sugar (starch), which release energy over a longer period of time.

Protein is an essential food component. The skin, muscles, bones, indeed all the body's organs are built with this. The hormones (or messenger substances), enzymes (base of cell metabolism), as well as the anti-bodies are all proteins in constant need of renewal. Thus it is important, that we don't absorb too much protein, but rather ensure that we utilize the best sources of protein. Too high protein intake especially animal protein means that we get too much saturated fat and cholesterol as well as releasing nitrogen, which is expelled via the kidneys with a lot of valuable minerals. In radical diets, one loses mainly fluids and body protein, which is gradually broken down and lost.

The fat in our diet serves mainly to store up energy in our body. Fat has twice as many calories as protein or carbohydrates and so, anyone wishing to lose weight, must not cut out fat completely, or essential fatty acids and fat-dissolving vitamins (A, D, E and K) cannot be utilized by the body. There are also different kinds of fat: Vegetable fats (e.g. cold-pressed oils) contain more essential fatty acids than animal fats (e.g. butter and lard).

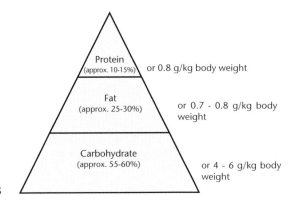

Diagram 17:
Pyramid of food products

7.1.2 Minerals and Vitamins

Minerals are the sparking **plugs of our metabolism,** enabling chemical reactions to take place in the body, as well as being important for conducting nerve impulses and also necessary for muscle contraction.

Vitamins are the **igniting sparks of our metabolism,** being an important component of the enzymes which steer carbohydrate and protein metabolic process in order (32).

Vitamins C and E are anti-oxidants to combat the free radicals. They protect us against Ultra-Violet rays, chemical pollution, burns and many types of cancer, as well as strengthening our immune system and prevent our arteries getting furred up (arterical calcification!). Vitamins C and E are equally important in preventing the build-up of collagen, which has its influence on the cellulite structure.

7.1.3 Water – The Basis of all Processes

Water lies at the root of all life processes, without which our organism cannot function at all. Human beings consist of up to 2/3 water, which accumulates within the cells, but also in the so-called extra-cellular space in between all the billions of body cells. Small children have a greater supply of body fluid viewed from a chemical point of view, old people have less, seen externally in a more dried-out skin. Water is more or less the nutrient solution for transporting various nutritional products and biosynthesis, although water is not just water. Water containing minerals and trace elements is indispensible for all one's metabolism. So that water in fruit and vegetables, in its complete physiologically-balanced state, is the most important source of the body's health. We are constantly and urgently reminded to drink enough regularly.

Doctors and food biologists recommend a daily intake of at least 2.5 litres of liquid. Whoever eats enough fruit can however reduce their amount of drink and can manage without mineral drinks during leisure sport, as these are not wonder drinks but synthetically produced isotonic drinks (31).

If you have put on a pound or two too much, then your body suffers from extra weight i.e. from water retection, because the **fatty tissues store up water like a sponge**, up to twice the amount of normal connective tissue. Typical signs of water retention (oedema) in addition to the well-known little cushions in problem areas, are swollen joints and, especially early in the morning, a swollen face with "puffy" eyes. The less fatty tissue, the less water it is able to collect, so we are not just talking about your figure but also about your health. It is well-known that fatty cells develop in early youth and remain fairly constant in number throughout one's life. The fatty deposits at one's stomach, on the arms, hips and thighs can be drained by certain natural products, and swellings in the face and joints can recede.

If you are overweight, the logical conclusion in its fullest sense of the word is that most of it is "superfluous".

The function of water

Water is a **means of dissolving nutrients** which can be absorbed into the blood via the gut.

Water is a **means of transporting** nutrients, oxygen and waste products to the excretary organs.

Water is a **building material** of which 2/3 appears in the tissues and only about 1/3 in the form of blood, lymph and tissue fluid.

Water is a **temperature gauge**, as for maintaining various body functions it is of great importance to human beings to have constant body temperature.

Water is one of the elixiers of life, the oldest beauty product in the world and the best kind of medicine, as water cleans from inside (31). People, who drink a lot of it ensure that their bodies are kept free of waste products and the body's waste and damaging substances are got rid of sooner. The very best creams have only limited effect if the skin is too dry – so – **drink yourself beautiful!**

What sort of water is effective?

Healing Water must come from underground springs and be filled at source. A further prerequisite: a high proprrotion of effective substances (e.g. sulphur, iodine, iron, fluoride) - there must be a scientifically recognized certificate to prove its healding qualities.

Spring Water must certainly come from a genuine underground spring and have drinking water qualities; but a minimum amount of minerals and trace elements is not necessarily required.

Table Water needs no special offical recognition, and can theoretically be produced by anyone. It is usually a mixture of drinking- and natural mineral water, which can be mixed with other ingredients or minerals.

Dieting with apple vinegar can support the weight-loosing process and indeed accelerate it. Apple vinegar encourages metabolism, enhances the body's basal metabolism together with body fat cumbustion. Although, on the one hand one's appetite is enhanced by apple vinegar, it has also been proved that a small glass of apple vinegar water between meals makes the stomach feel pleasantly full, which reduces the appetite. It is recommended that initially one takes 1 glass of water with 2 teaspoonfuls of apple vinegar and 1 teaspoon of honey three times a day in small sips. Ensure that you choose good quality organic apple vinegar. Around 20 minerals and trace elements can be found in apple vinegar e.g. potassium, copper, fluoride, calcium, chloride, iron, calium, magnesium, sulphur, silicium, boron...

Apple vinegar can help get rid of fat, helps the organism absorb vitamins, minerals and trace elements, drains the system, encourages the excretion of waste and poisonous substances, improves renal functions, regulates the acid and base products' supply and supports the functioning of the nerve cells. Despite of all this, make sure that you continue to feel well after the recommended mixture. After a week, you only need to take this effective mixture once a day. The water-vinegar proportion can be adjusted by mixing only one teaspoon of apple vinegar with a glass of lukewarm water at room temperature (14).

Nutritional recommendations

- Use at best only natural food products with high nutritional content.
- Lower your fat, sugar, alcohol, salt and meat consumption as well as milk products with a high fat content.
- Eat slowly and chew thoroughly.
- Eat a balanced diet.
- Eat enough to satisfy the body's needs (but not the soul's as well!).
- Don't omit any meals; better to have 5-6 small meals than two huge meals.
- Moderation in all things "it is the amount that counts".
- Eat healthy foods at parties first, after which you may enjoy some sweet things.
- Take your last meal before 7 pm and afterwards only fresh fruit and vegetables.

Hundreds of medical prohibitions and moral rules promise a long and happy life. However, without the little sins there is no great pleasure.

Already as in 1993 the Berlin sociologist Hagen Kühn enlarged the German language by the term „Healthismus" (healthism) and he warns of the incessent bombardement with health advices and codes of conduct. Guilty feelings create heavy and illness causing stress. Only to know about the problems does not motivate. Preventive measures can only work if being fun and being felt as pleasure sensation. There is no quality of life without the little sins like coffein, alcohol or sweets, all enjoyed moderately of course (18).

7.2 Energy Requirements

Every person needs a different mixture of energy, which can come from one's basic turnover, or one's turnover at work or in one's leisure time.

Basic turnover: the amount of energy needed to maintain one's general body functions.

Basic turnover

Women
between 20 and 34 = body weight x 21.6
between 35 and 50 = body weight x 19.2

Men
between 20 and 34 = body weight x 24
between 35 and 50 = body weight x 21.6

Chart 5: Basic turnover

Another way of calculating one's calorific needs:

Men: (body weight x 1 kcal/hour x 24)
Women: (body weight x 0.9 kcal/hour x 24)

Work turnover: the amount of extra calories required depends on the level of activity of the work; – 500 kcal/day for easy work; – 1000 kcal/day for a medium level of work, 1500 kcal/day for hard or the hardest type of work. A white-collar worker (e.g. sitting at a desk) saves energy, whereas a competitive sportsman "wastes energy".

Leisure turnover: energy should be converted by means of sporting activities i.e. good for one's health: optimum 7 kcal/kg.

Example: a man, 32 years old, 80 kg.

basic turnover:	80 kg x 24	= 1920 calories
work turnover:	sitting activity	= 500 calories
leisure turnover:	80 kg x 7 kcal/kg	= 560 calories

So the calorific requirement of a 32 year-old man, who mainly engages in a sedentary occupation, but does sport regularly is 1920 + 500 + 560 = 2980 calories.

The calorific need is proportionally greater, the longer and more intensively one trains and the more muscle groups are worked in anaerobic way. The fatty tissues can only be burnt off with the aid of oxygen. Endurance sports like aerobics, jogging, cycling, long-distance running are the best ways of reducing weight.

7.3 Anti-Cellulite Substances

The first step in getting rid of orange skin is the change of one's dietary habits. It is only possible to maintain a healthy diet if we feed our bodies with a variety of good and healthy food products in the right balance and proportion.

The following food stuffs can reduce water and waste products in our tissues:

Pineapples	(bromelain, biotin, vitamin E, vitamin B_{12})
Potatoes	(potassium, vitamin C etc)
Avocados	(potassium, magnesium, vitamin D, B_6 etc)
Millet	(silicium, iron, magnesium, fluoride etc)

Broccoli	(potassium, zinc, copper, vitamins C and A etc)
Barley	(silicium, zinc, selenium, magnesium etc)
Sauerkraut	(potassium, copper, vitamin C etc)
Mushrooms	(potassium, copper, selenium, iron etc)
Bananas	(potassium, silicium, magnesium, vitamin B_6 etc)
Spinach	(potassium, calcium, magnesium, vitamins A and C, folic acid etc)

7.3.1 The Functioning of these Substances

The valuable substances contained in fruit, vegetables, nuts, pulses and wholemeal products keep our innate body immune system and other organs in trim in a perfectly natural way.

Biotin	important for an attractive skin, hair, nails, blood sugar level, muscle cell function (e.g. pineapples).
Bromelain	miracle enzyme – improves the circulation, prevents inflammation and relaxes the muscles (e.g. pineapples).
Potassium	helps to get rid of surplus water from the tissues, regulates (as an opponent of sodium) the body's water supply, ensures that the tissues get rid of surplus salt. Potassium is our secret weapon in the fight against cellulite (e.g. potatoes).
Copper	good for making the connective tissues firmer and more flexible (e.g. mushrooms).
Magnesium	activates many enzymes (e.g. avocados).
Selenium	guards against the free radicals (e.g. barley).
Silicium	a "scaffold-building" substance with which all living organisms build up their bones, teeth, "armour", skin, hair and nails. It also strengthens the connective tissue (e.g. millet).
Vitamin D	indispensible for strengthening of bones and teeth (vitamin D is made of cholesterol in the human organism). Cholesterol in the skin is turned into vitamin D by the sun, so the vitamin D level in the body is directly related to how much sun we get and cannot be regulated by what we eat.
Zinc	guards against the free radicals and is important for the building up of connective tissues (e.g. broccoli).

7.4 Diets

With the term "diet", the Greek definition does not only mean how we feed ourselves, but also one's whole **attitude to life i.e. physically as well as psychologically**. Diet (diaita = way of life) comprises the basis for a sensible way of life, which includes adequate diet, sensible physical activity and the avoidance of damaging patterns of behaviour like smoking, alcohol abuse and drug-taking. In more recent years, the term "diet" has been confined to reducing one's calorific intake.

In Germany, 30-40% of the population suffer from overweight (adiposity), which stems first and foremost from an inappropriate diet and the wrong sort of habits.
Overweight can lead to other negative results: e.g. psychological disorders (disorders in one's self-esteem), heart and circulatory diseases, diabetes mellitus type II (blood sugar disease), additional weight on one's supporting and mobility structure (backache), formation of tumors etc. The mortality rate also increases with overweight.

A radical diet implies stress for our organism and in stress situations, massive amounts of stress hormones e.g. **Cortisol** are released. The energy dispensers, glucose suppliers in the muscles and liver are qickly drained. Smaller amounts of energy are prepared as fatty acids by the fat cells, but these act as energy reserves and are of great importance in times of great need.

They are mobilized in stress situations, but as soon as nourishment is re-introduced, they return to the adipocytes. If food is withheld over a larger period of time, the body forms sugar by dissolving its innate protein, mainly drawn from the muscles. Human beings have a fat regulating device, the so-called "**adipostate**", situated in the hypothalamus (part of the interbrain) next to the temperature-regulating centre. This adipstate ensures a constant balance of fat within the organism.

Leptin hormones, found in the fatty tissues, let the adipostate know what the fat level is (current level). During times of radical dieting, this regulating device is permanently on "alarm". The organism tries to conserve as much energy as possible in this period of time and the person only thinks about eating. Peace and quiet returns when the fat cells are full up agian and the adipostate has reached its set value. Often only half the amount of time is needed to fill the fat dispensers, because the basic turnover is less in a time of emergency, which the body notes for next time, so the well-known yo-yo effect is there.

All attempt to lose weight by dieting alone fail in the majority of cases.

Four reasons for not going on a radical diet:

1. **Strict diets** (under 1200 kcal per day) reduce water, fat and muscle protein. This emergency situation, due to a reduced calorie intake, forces the body to turn to its own reserves. Our organism does not only burn fat, but also vital protein **(own, personal cannibalism)**.

   If more protein is got rid of than fat, than the body's composition deteriorates. The human organism has no protein reserves of its own. So, when dieting, the prime aim should be to reduce the amount of fat in the body and not to lose any functional or structural protein.

   During the long kind of diets, the end effect is a greater percentage of fat than before. Muscle-building training can considerably reduce the muscular decline of organic protein during dieting and thus look after the muscles.

2. **Dramatic reduction of one's calorific intake** forces the body to reduce its energy output. A human's metabolism is programmed to a certain extent for survival in times of emergency, the so-called **"survival syndrome"**. The whole organism switches over to minimum cumbustion or "just ticking over".

   Metabolism can still take place slowly. In this kind of stress situation, the body releases a flow of stress hormones (cortisol), because it is concerned with its survival. This cortisol gives the body glucose from its protein depots especially from the muscles and the heart.

   The body's own proteins produce the largest amount of energy. The free fatty acids are partly mobilized from the fat depots, but the highest proportion circulates in the blood and are stored away again as soon as the hunger phase is over. After certain substances have been got rid of, over-compensation takes place i.e. the body does not only compensate for its loss, but also builds up more substances than before (protection for another hunger phase).

3. Anyone who is always trying different diets, can count on the **yo-yo effect** (oscillating body weight). Because of the lack of success he/she is then not only psychologically but also physically frustrated.

One's metabolism suffers negative training effects, as it learns more and more to switch over to conserving energy and then to store energy faster and faster when the dieting is over. The glucose gained from dissolving the muscles raises the insulin level. This, in turn, produces increased stress, which can lead to permanent stress. In the end the fasting person loses less and less weight and puts on weight faster and faster.

4. "Miracle diets" are constantly sold to us in many woman's magazines, as suggestions for diets always get a good press. Most diets have one thing in common: they aim towards a **one-sided, reduced food intake**, which brings quick results to start with.

The monotony and one-sidedness can however, lead to serious **risks to one's health.** The body's metabolism gets out of balance. The bones become brittle, the skin loses its tone, the muscles their elasticity and the construction of new cells in the connective tissues is impaired. A further disadvantage of radical dieting is an increased risk of infection. So, the end result is: gain of new weight but loss of health.

Unfortunately, in the area of weight reduction, innumerable pointless types of dieting have developed in recent years. There is no balanced food choice in many of these diets and so many are in fact health-damaging. Various bottle-necks in the supply of food makes it impossible to recommend anything. Many theories are impossible to prove scientifically.

8 Stress Management

We live our lives between two related poles: activity-rest, work-leisure, tension-relaxation, sadness-joy etc. Only when a certain balance is achieved between both poles do we feel really well in the fullest sense of the word.

Relaxation which reduces stress helps to minimize nervousness, irritability, inner unrest and overloading. Relaxation is a whole lot more than hygiene for the soul. The close relationship between body and spirit is apparent when we are in a relaxed state. When stress hormones are released, we find ourselves in a state of acute awareness, which helps us to think more clearly and quickly. As soon as this emotional stress has been removed, our system is inclined to work more against us than for us. Any disorder in the system of the human organism automatically leads to a further chain reaction in the whole body. Stress and tension can lead to cellulite, because all the body's important functions change when tense or anxious: we breathe less deeply, our disgestion becomes sluggish, our circulation weaker and our glandular functions are affected.

All in all, this disbalances the organism and prepares the ground for cellulite. The amino acids (protein) are removed from the body during a state of permanent emotional stress and burnt off as "escapist" fuel. So, a lot of people lose weight when they are exposed to stress for a long time. The suprarenal glands, which produce amongst other things adrenalin, noradrenalin and cortisol, likewise regulate the body's water supply.

If the suprarenal gland is disturbed, then there is a disbalance in the sodium-potassium balance. Shallow breathing hinders cell metabolism and often causes tiredness. The blood vessels constrict which, consequently prevents a flow of blood to the body's extremities.

Stress produces stress. Changes in the body's processes due to stress can lead directly to cellulite.

Positive stress (eustress) released by endurance- or strength training makes us more resistent, so that we can overcome **negative stress (distress)**.

There are many forms of relaxation e.g. Jakobson's progressive muscle relaxation, general breathing relaxation, a journey through the body etc. It is immaterial which method you choose, as long as you reach your main goal i.e. the easing of states of tension and the restoration of a pleasant physical and mental feeling of peace and contentment. We can see how closely-related body and soul are for example by looking at tension in the skeletal muscles when a human being is emotionally overloaded.

8.1 The Positive Effects of Relaxation Training

Relaxation training done regularly can bring about the following effects:

- Reduction of muscular tension, nervousness and restlessness
- Improvement in concentration
- Reduction of stress
- Getting rid of fear (e.g. fear of exams)
- Speeding up of physical and psychological regeneration
- Soothing pain
- Encouraging calm, taking things easy and enhancing the feeling of contentment
- Lowering of breathing and heart rate
- Feeling of warmth and heaviness
- Expanding depth of breathing
  …

8.2 Relaxation Methods

There are several ways of relaxing and each of us should work out their own individual strategy for relaxation. One differentiates between procedures under **one's own control or controlled by someone else**. Massage and hypnosis belong in the latter category. Methods which you can control yourself can again be sub-divided into the **"naive"**, which cannot be learnt systematically and are not generally transferrable (e.g. walking, reading, listening to music etc) and the **"scientific"**, where one follows a course of teaching (e.g. Jacobson's progessive muscle relaxation, autogenic training, yoga etc).

JACOBSON'S progressive relaxation

In German-speaking countries, this method is usually called deep muscular relaxation (TME). The key features of the JACOBSON method are tension and relaxation. Tension is prime importance to JACOBSON, indeed vital, as tension in terms of muscles contracting enables all our movements and human activity. However, if it exceeds a certain limit, various disorders occur in the human organism.

JACOBSON wishes to get rid of any remaining tension in the body by muscular contraction. By using the two opposing poles of contraction and decontraction, anyone can feel how a clenched fist slowly loosens up and the fingers relax as they open. The sense of deep relaxation should spread progessively by learning how to systematically tense and then relax individual groups of muscles.

In my opinion, this is one of the easiest and most efficient relaxation methods, which I have seen to be effective with all ages of paritcipants.

An example for when you are leading a group:
Note:
- Each exercise can be repeated twice.
- ... denotes a rest of 10-15 secs.
- The tension can last beween 5-10 secs.

Exercise: Relaxing the arms

"Adopt a position as comfortable as possible - loosen up the tension in arms and legs. Relax as much as you can".

"Clench your right fist. Slowly but continually increase the pressure. Your fist is getting harder. Feel the tension in your right arm, in your underarm, ... And now relax. Loosen the fingers of your right hand and sense the pleasant feeling of relaxation. Let all tension go and feel how the relaxation spreads your right arm and throughout the rest of your body... Now do the same with your left hand. Clench your left fist, whilst the rest of your body relaxes. Clench your fist more firmly and feel the pressure... And then relax again. Sense and enjoy the difference...

Now clench both hands. Increase the pressure slowly but continually – the fingers become hard and the underarms are very tense. Feel the pressure... and relax. Loosen your fingers and feel the relaxation... Now raise your underarms and pull your arms closer to your body. Tense the muscles in your arms, increase the pressure and note the feelings of tension... Now let your arms go again, relax and feel the difference. Let the relaxation spread further... Now turn your hands over, so that your palms are facing upwards and press your hands and arms dowmwards towards the ground, firmly enough to sense tension in your muscles... And then relax. Your arms are again in a comfortable position. Let your arms relax further... Now settle yourself into comfortable relaxation in your arms, to relaxing without any tension at all... Even if you think your arms are now fully relaxed, try and loosen them a bit further. Your arms are getting heavier and warmer. They relax more and more ... "

Exercise: Relaxing the face and shoulders

Remain in your quiet and comfortable position. All your muscles are heavy and relaxed... Raise your eyebrows and frown. Increase the feeling of tension... then release the tension. Relax your eyebrows, your scalp, then your forehead. Feel how your skin becomes smoother, the more you relax... Now close your eyes. Close them tightly, but not so that the pressure becomes uncomfortable. Feel the pressure... and release the tension. The eyes remain shut. Feel the relaxation...

Now bite your teeth together firmly and tense your jaw. Concentrate on the tension in your lower jaw... Loosen up your jaw again and enjoy this relaxed feeling... Now tense your tips. Press them against each other and feel the tension... Now release the tension again and feel how the relaxed feeling spreads across your face. Your hips, jaw, throat, eyes and forehead all become relaxed. The relaxation extends further... Now turn your attention to your neck muscles. Push your head backwards and feel the tension at the back of your neck. Roll your neck in slow motion to the right and feel the change of tension. Then push your head to the left and feel how the sense of tension changes... Then let your head return to a comfortable position. Feel the pleasant sense of release. Enjoy the peace... Now press your chin against your chest and feel a slight closeness... Then release the tension and sense the freedom. Let the relaxation continue... Now pull up your shoulders very firmly. Maintain this tension... Let your shoulders fall again loosely and sense the release. Back of the neck and shoulders relax. Let the relaxation spread right through your shoulders as far as the back muscles. Relax the back of your neck and your face and feel how deep relaxation spreads further. It goes on and on..."

Exercise: Relaxing the trunk

"Get into a comfortable position. Loosen up as well as you can. You are breathing freely and easily. Feel how relaxation increases just like breathing out. Now breathe in deeply, so that stomach and chest are arched and hold your breath ... and then breathe out. Let your stomach and rib cage relax; the air flows out automatically.

As the breath pours out, notice how you continue to relax. Enjoy the relaxation ... it spreads across your stomach, your chest, your shoulders, your back. Enjoy the relaxation ... Now tense your stomach muscles, as you push your stomach outwards. Make your stomach muscles firm and hard ... and then relax. Loosen your muscles and feel the pressure ... Now relax. Loosen your stomach muscles again.

Then pull your stomach in again. Maintain this tension ... Press your stomach outwards. Maintain this tension as well and sense the differences ... And now relax your stomach muscles. The tension disappears and relaxation increases. Each time you breathe out, feel the increasing relaxation in your rib cage and in your stomach; give in to the feeling of relaxation.

All the tension in your body loosens up more ... Now concentrate on your back. Support yourself with shoulders. Arch your upper body upwards. Increase the tension in your back and in your shoulder muscles ... then get into a comfortable position again. Loosen up ... Let the pleasant feeling of relaxation extend further. In your shoulders, your arms and your face the relaxation increases. You relax more and more ... ."

Exercise: Relaxing the legs

"Stay relaxed and enjoy the inner peace ... Now stretch your legs out in front of you and tense your bottom and thighs. Increase the tension ... and then relax. Sense the difference between tension and relaxation ... Press your feet and toes downwards, away from your face, so that your calf muscles are tense. Feel the tension ... then relax your feet and calves. Sense the release of tension ... . Now pull your legs nearer to your body and put the soles of your feet flat on the ground. Then raise your heels. Increase the tension ... Loosen up your heels and legs again. Sense the release of tension in your legs. This time bend your feet in the direction of your face. Bring your toes right up and sense the tension in your shins ... Relax and bring your legs back into a comfortable position. Get ready for deep relaxation. Relax your feet, your calves, your shins, your knees, all your leg muscles, your bottom, your hips. Feel the heaviness of your lower body, whilst the relaxation continues ..."

Exercise: Relaxing the whole body

"Stay in your quiet and comfortable position. All your muscles are fully relaxed ... Concentrate on your stomach. The wall of stomach rises and falls by itself. Extend the relaxation to your lower spine. Let yourself go more and more. Feel the relaxation. It extends further across your back, your chest, your shoulders and arms down to your fingertips. Relax completely ... Let go off all tension in your throat. Relax your neck, your jaw and the rest of your facial muscles. You are breathing freely and quietly. Your loosely closed eyes deepen the relaxation further ... Enjoy the inner peace and being sunk into yourself ... In this state of total relaxation, you are not even capable of moving a muscle in your body. Think of the effort it would take to raise your right arm ... Check whether the very thought of this causes any tension your shoulders or arms ... Then, decide not to raise your arm. Remain in a state of peaceful, deep relaxation.

Return

"If you want to finish this exercise, take back the feeling of heaviness, by suddenly pulling your arms towards you and then stretching them out. Stretch yourself out, breathe in and out deeply, open your eyes. You feel at ease, refreshed and agreeably calm (3)."

8.3 Tips for Relaxation Training

The following principles should be born in mind during relaxation training:

- A comfortable position for relaxing in supine at best for the JACOBSON method.
- Wear warm and comfortable clothes.
- Tune in to the relaxation (e.g. eyes shut, breathe in deeply, correct your position, let your thoughts float away ...).
- Emphasize relaxed breathing (the stomach wall rises and falls).
- Eliminate any disturbance factors from outside.
- Draw attention to negative associations, fear unrest before relaxing and possibly "take back" the relaxation, because it cannot be forced, but one must simply give way to this condition.
- Feelings of heaviness and warmth are signs of total relaxation.
- "Taking back" or "Returning" means activating the circulation again: Clenching one's fists, tensing arm and leg muscles, opening one's eyes, breathing deeply, stretching and lolling about.
- It is a good idea to learn about relaxation techniques on a course with a qualified teacher.
- Relaxation music can have a favourable effect on the "letting go".
- Sleep is the best anti-stress therapy, consciously shut out feelings of fear, anxiety and worries when you go to bed.

Regular relaxation training is the best and most effective miracle drug in a universal type of medicine without side effects. Arrange an appointment for it regularly with yourself!

9 Skin Care

Research laboratories have been trying for years to find products to counteract the ageing process of our skin. Many anti-cellulite products have since appeared on the market in the form of cream, gel, lotion, oil etc which always have the same objective i.e. to activate the flow of lymphatic fluid, to boost cell metabolism and stimulate one's circulation.

Body care does not just mean putting cream on your skin, but also massaging it. For example, it could be a rolling and pinching massage with the fingers, massage with a roller, luffa glove, brush or electrical gadgets. You can only seriously do something against cellulite by daily massage.

9.1 Cosmetics

A smooth-skinned body always has a youthful and attractive effect, even if the figure is somewhat fuller. On the other hand, if the skin loses its smoothness, winkles and cellulite appear. After losing weight too quickly, too much sun-bathing or even naturally as one gets older, the skin loses its smoothness. Research laboratories try all the time to find new ways of penetrating further into the skin. Scientists have found out that 0.1% of the skin's surface is not covered by horny layer, because openings for fat and sweat come out here. At these points, substances like vitamins A, E and C can penetrate the skin which help with better circulation and also the getting rid of waste products from the tissues.

The manufacturers of anti-cellulite products are automatically convinced that their own products are effective, I quote: "...but now there is a product available to all women, which maintains the body's youthful firmness." These are comfortable methods, which don't take much time or trouble to apply and their dispensing is developed accordingly. The objective is always the same: to speed up cell metabolism, to accelerate the formation of "scaffolding matter" (collagen) and to activate the activity of the lymph glands, so that waste and damaging materials can be got rid of quickly.

The following **products** are used in the cosmetic industry:

Ginko – a substance form the Ginkgobiloba tree is often used in conjunction with coffein and is supposed to support fat disposal and metabolism.

Guarana – is supposed to enhance basic cell metabolism and accelerate fat disposal in the cells.

Hydroxic acid (AHA = Alpha-Hydro-Acids) – are supposed to stimulate the formation of new cells and make the skin far receptive for anti-cellulite substances.

Coffein should break up chains of fat in the tissues and, when combined with Cola-nut extract, should help speed up flow of lymphatic fluid.

Ruskus should strengthen the walls of the vessels and improve lymphatic circulation.

Nicotinic acid promotes a warming effect in thermo-creams, which encurage a widering of the blood vessels and thus speed up the removal of water and waste porducts.

Sorrel root is reputed to be a good diuretic.

Silicium is a mineral which builds firm and stable vessels and is thus in part resonsible for the firmness of the connective tissues.

Before a cosmetic product or medicine comes onto the market, it must undergo rigorous tests by the manufacturer. "Live" tests are done on the skin of certain willing "guinea pig" people. The results are thus subjective and can be either positive or negative depending on how they are produced (e.g. as gel, cream, lotion etc) and many other factors. It is virtually impossible to give an objective statement about their effect on one's skin.

As all anti-cellulite preparations contain skin-protecting and lubricating substances, the cosmetic effect on the surface of the skin is undisputed. You will only see results if applied daily. However, to achieve real and lasting success, you need to combine these products with massage, sport, the right kind of diet and a certain amount of discipline.

9.2 Massage

To optimize the effort of many anti-cellulite substances, we recommend a simple but very effective purification supporting massage. Waste product disposal in the tissues is accelerated by gentle pressure of the hands or certain apparatus and so the lymphatic system and blood circulation are activated and cell tissue activity improved.

Massage can be done with just the hands and is regarded as particularly effective.

Massage with a fairly hard brush or cellulite roller can improve the circulation and make the skin visibly softer. But one must not forget that the be all and end all is daily massage.

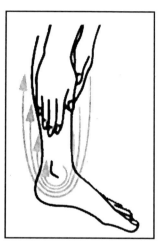

Diagram 18: Massaging the lower leg

An example of massage:
1. *The lower leg:*
    clasp your ankle with both hands and massage in increasingly big circles up to the knee.

2. *The tigh:*
    clasp your knee with both hands and massage the thigh in increasingly big circles towards the top.

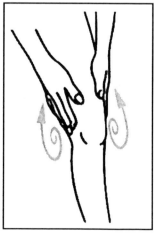

Diagram 19: Massaging the tigh

3. *Rolling massage of the thigh:*
   clasp the outside of your thigh with both hands and knead the bulge outwards.

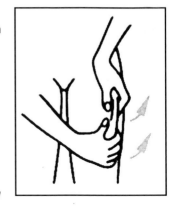

Diagram 20: Rolling massage of the thigh

4. Drainage points:
   clasp your thigh with both hands above the knee. Place your thumbs at the same time about ten times lightly on the inner thigh and move them upwards slowly.

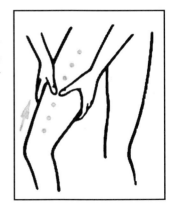

Diagram 21: Drainage points massage

5. Base of the tigh and bottom:
   massage in a circle from the hip downwards and then up again completely incorporating your bottom.

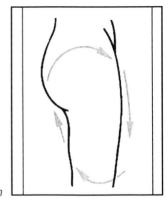

Diagram 22: Massaging the thigh and bottom

Another way of massaging places endangered by cellulite is massage with a **nobbly ball**. The following exercises promote the circulation in your bottom and thigh areas and thus help combat cellulite.

Ex.:
Sitting on the ball. Do circular movements with your pelvis (10-20 to the right and 10-20 to the left). The back remains straight.

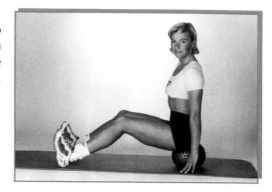

Ex.:
Sitting on the ball. Roll the ball under your bottom and thigh muscles. Put your arms behind your body and keep your back straight.

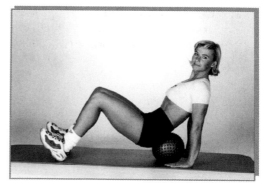

Ex.:
Side position. The ball is under the thigh, then roll backwards and forwards on the ball towards the knee and hip.

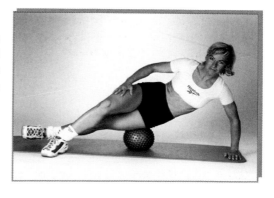

10 Additional Methods

There is a whole range of beauty treatments, and yet a woman's skin and tissues all react differently. A smooth face, well-formed bust, flat stomach and slim hips are what every woman would like, but this is seldom realistic in practice.

- If diets and anti-ninkle creams do not work in the long run, then the magic word is "Cosmetic surgery" i.e. beauty on demand.
  Plastic surgery is being used more and more. Liposuction (sucking off fat) has spurred many women onto working towards their ideal figure. From a technical point of view, the problem area is marked out first. Then under partial of full anaesthetic, the surgeon injects a special solution of cooking salt and adrenalin, which reduces swelling and bleeding as well as it is building up the tissue. Using small 2-3 mm cuts, little cannulas are inserted by which the sub-cutaneous fat in the designated areas is sucked away. The area operated on is then bound up with a pressure bandage.

Advantage: Cushions of fat anywhere in the body can be modelled and you can have your body proportions altered as you wish. The operation is done as an outpatient and lasts between three and five hours.

Disadvantage: bleeding afterwards, swelling and sudden bleeding if the regulations are not adhered to. You need to wear a corset or bodice for at least four weeks.

Price: Starts at around £500.

- **Lypolysis with low electric current** is another way of dealing with cellulite. Very fine needles up to 15 cm long are pushed under the skin parallel to the surface, and then connected to electrical apparatus by electrodes. The metabolism in the fatty cells improves, water in the tissues is got rid of via the kidneys. The treatment lasts for about 45 min. After about eight sessions at weekly intervals, the skin looks more even.

Advantage: a slight but insignificant amount of cellulite disappears.

Disadvantage: the effect does not last long time.

Price: about £80 per treatment.

- The latest form of therapy to make the sub-cutaneous tissue smoother and reduce its size is the so-called **"Liponic Sculpting"** using a computer. The treatment head of the equipment, which consists of two big flat rolls between which a powerful vacuum is built up, moves over the affected parts of the body. The aim is to reduce liquid in the fatty cells, supported by the rolling massage.

Advantage: extreme forms of cellulite can be treated; at the most, you can achieve two clothing sizes smaller.

Disadvantage: this is a very costly method as initial treatment is necessary twice a week for 45 minutes each time. To maintain results, you need to be treated once a month.

Price: about £70 per treatment.

- By the **deep warming** method, the affected areas are bound up with heatable elastic bandages. They warm the tissues to a depth of 3 cm with the aid of ultra-red rays. The body is warmed up to around 40-42 °C. This accelerates metabolism and water can be washed out of the tissues.

Advantage: if repeated enough times, considerable results can be achieved.

Disadvantage: not advisable from a medical point of view if suffering from circulatory problems, metabolic disorders, weak veins, kidney or thyroid problems. At least ten one-hour sessions.

Price: around £17.

- Cellulite treatment with **electric stimulation** belongs in the hands of the professionals. All electric stimulation apparatus is geared to moving the muscles in the problem areas positively. The theory behind this states: during the movements in the muscles caused by the electrical stimulations, energy is being used up. This energy is supplied by the fat cells round about. The procedure is simple: two or more electrodes are fixed to the areas to be treated with elastic bands. Electrocables are fixed to the electrodes, which are connected to the apparatus. By pressing a button electric current is applied directly to the muscles.

Advantage: the gentle vibration has a relaxing effect. There are electrical stimulation devices you can use at home.

Disadvantage: counter-productive with varicose veins and for inflammatory and feverish conditions, as well as open wounds and skin injuries. The treatment also has little effect on flabby connective tissue.

Price: About £700 if you want to buy an electrical stimulation device for use at home (13).

- In extreme cases of cellulite, the lymphatic system is usually also disturbed. The lymphatic fluid is normally kept moving by muscular activity, and it sinks into the tissue if there is insufficient movement. **Lymph drainage** aims at restoring the flow, so that liquid can be got rid of. During lymph drainage, one is massaged with gentle smoking and light circular pumping movements along the lymph vessels into direction of lymph nodes. To be sure of successful treatment, put yourself in the hands of a qualified therapist or beauty specialist. But you can help youself at home. The new anti-cellulite massage apparatus, which has proved a success on beauty farms and can now be used at home is called **"Cellesse"** made by **PHILIPS**. "Cellesse" works on the lymph drainage theory. The skin together with sub-cutaneous tissue is lifted, massaged and the fluid then removed. "Cellesse" is available in electrical shops, perfumeries, drug stores, and from sanitary specialists.

Advantage: a natural and gentle method. The "Cellesse" equipment is easy to use. A comprehensive information brochure enables you to massage yourself easily.

Disadvantage: conter-productive if suffering from an injection, you have a temperature or you have a tendency to thrombosis.

Price: around £13 per treatment.
"Cellesse" from PHILIPS costs £100.

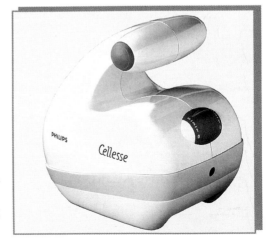

Since time immemorial it has been well known that **water** has excellent effects on the skin tissue. Stimuli by changing temperature (hot and cold showers) are as well recommended as taking baths with additional substances (e.g. salt- or algae-baths) to stimulate the blood circulation or soft water massages to decongest the tissue. Sponge-downs with **ice** or **vingar water** keep your skin smooth.

There are many other "professional ways" of "ironing out" the dents and flabs, but there is not as yet any scientifically proved research into individual methods. Beauty institutes record good results, but the individual chances of success vary enormously. Anyone who thinks to rescue a relationship from the rocks with a well-formed bottom or to regain one's necessary self-confidence, is more in need of psychotherapy than of an appointment with a beauty surgeon. So: act rather than operate.

If you do not do any specific endurance or strength training and feed yourself properly, then you can only expect short-term results; because **true beauty starts from inside.**

Part III

ANTI-CELLULITE TRAINING IN PRACTICE

11 Endurance Training

The most important load intensity control gauge for endurance sports is your heart rate. You can choose between indoor and outdoor sports, depending on your particular interest and the weather. Sports shops offer a wide range of heart and circulation apparatus (bike hometrainer, step machine, ...) by which you can "power out" at home. Heart and circulation training on a home trainer can be supported by rhythmic music, but you need a lot of willpower to get yourself onto your bike every or every alternate day. The alternative is to visit a club or fitness studio where you have to pay a fee and keep to a fixed time. This way it is possibly easier to keep it up longer because the motivation and fun is greater in a group. Having a friend who also enjoys gymnastics is another motivating factor. Choose a type of sport which you can also do in bad weather.

The intensity of various endurance sports:

High: fast jogging, intensive aerobics and step aerobics, riding a mountain bike, intensive ergometer training (bike, rowing apparatus, stepper etc), skipping, beach volleyball, rowing, tennis.

Medium: moderate aerobics and step aerobics, ergometer training, swimming, cross-country skiing, aqua training, mountaineering, inline-skating.

Low: walking, golf.

Endurance running (jogging) ensures maximum burning off of calories and other healthy adjustments with a minimum amount of load and in a minumum amount of time. People who are obese or who have orthopaedic problems in the large-jointed areas like knees and hips should find some alternative forms of training for losing weight like swimming or cycling.

In health-orientated endurance training you can choose between minimal and optimal programmes.

Minimal programme:
The aim of this programme is to achieve notable results which have a positive effect on one's health.

The minimal programme should take up a total of **about 60 minutes per week,** whereby it is better to train **three times per week** for 20 minutes (mondays, wednesdays and fridays) than to do 60 minutes all at one go. The gap of the 7 days until the next training session is too big. Increasing the performance level with untrained people is high to begin with, but if you do not increase your range of training, you reach a peak in your performance after a few weeks and do not improve any further.

Optimal programme:
This programme is made up of **three to four hours training per week,** divided into **four or five units** and where large groups of muscles are worked on (jogging, cycling etc). Here, an increase in the range of training would raise orthopaedic load.

The training should be within the anaerobic area (see chapter 6.1.3) and there is no point in training excessively, because this can have a negative effect on your health.

You should take care especially what sort of shoes you are wearing and these are characterized by cushioning for the balls of your feet and at the heels which protects the joints.

12 Muscle Strengthening

Strengthened muscles give our body an attractive shape and have a toning and firming effect. Good muscle tone is vital for problem-free blood and lymphatic fluid circulation, as well as for the optimum running of all our body functions. The larger the mass of muscle, the more "combustion stores" we have at our disposal, which speeds up our metabolism and makes the burning of calories more efficient.

You need to have patience, as shaping up your body takes a long time and you do not see any positive changes from regular training until a few weeks later. Avoid overdoing it, which only stresses your body, otherwise you will not make it to the end of your period of training.

- Train **four to five times per week to begin with,** until you are satisfied with the result.

- To **maintain your fitness,** you should **train three times per week.**

- Choose at least two exercises out of three from the available exercises. Amount: 10-30 repetitions, 2-5 sets with a rest every 1-2 minutes.

- At the start of any fitness unit, have a **warming-up session** to loosen your muscles and prevent injury.

- You can train more effectively by using **additional apparatus,** but you can equally well do the exercises without apparatus, but ensuring that you tense your muscles.

If you train regularly, you do not only build up your muscles and get rid of fat, but also your skin, bottom and legs become smoother and the connective tissue firmer, so that cellulite does not have a chance!

12.1 Arm and Shoulder Muscles

Strengthening the arm muscles is of great importance both from an aesthetic and a health point of view. The biceps muscle and its antagonist, the triceps muscle, are found in the upper arm and can be strengthened individually. They are also trained during many other exercises (e.g. rowing, latissimus-pulling etc....).

Much more important are the muscles in the shoulder joint, as this has hardly any boney guidance and must therefore be protected by muscles. A very important muscle in this area is the deltoid muscle (M. deltadeus) which steers the arm sideways (abduction) and is involved in movements forwards and backwards as well as inner and outer rotating.

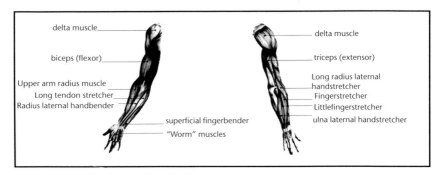

Diagram 23. Shoulder blade muscles (modified according to GEIGER, SCHMID, 1997, p.19)

Ex. with physio bar

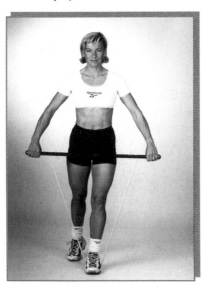 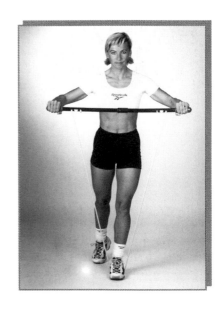

Starting position:
In a stepping position with legs slightly bent. Arms at the side of the body with elbows slightly bent.

Final position:
Arms are lifted horizontally out in front of you.

Ex.: with physiotape

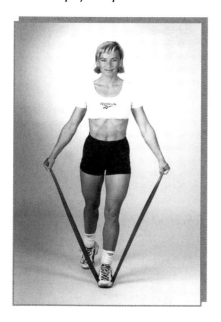

Starting position:
In a stepping position with arms stretched out to the side.

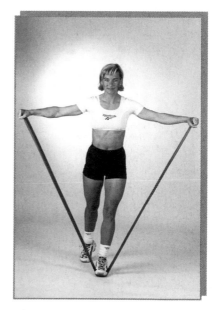

Final position:
Arms are lifted horizontally and sideways with palms facing the ceiling.

Ex.: with physio tube toner

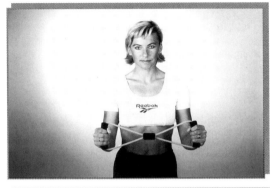

Starting position:
In a stepping position with arms bent at 90°, the toner is held in front of the body and put under tension.

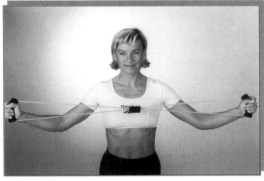

Final position 1:
The arms are taken to the side with the back of the hands pointing backwards.

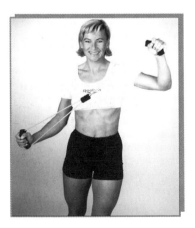

Final position 2:
The arms are placed diagonally.

Ex.: with physiotape

Starting position:
In a stepping position with both arms bent at the elbows and back of the hands facing the floor.

Final position:
Arms are bent with a slight outwards rotation in the elbow joint.

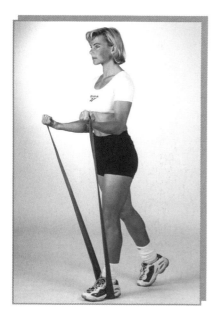

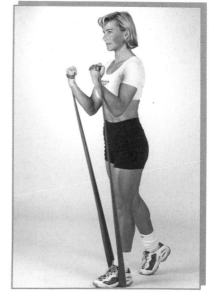

Ex.: with physio tube basic

Starting position:
In a stepping position, put your right leg in front of you and anchor the physio tube basic. Bend your left arm and put your elbow behind you.

Final position:
Stretch your left arm down behind you keeping your elbow at the back.

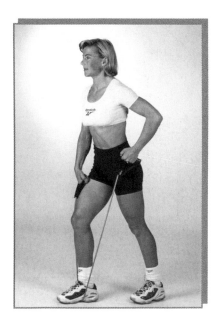

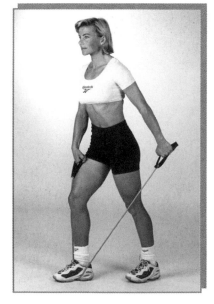

Ex.: press-ups

Starting position:
Quadruped position. Bend your lower leg putting the weight of your upper body forwards. Tense your stomach keeping your head in line with your spine and both arms slightly bent.

Final position:
Arms are stretched out.

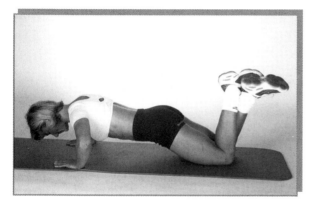

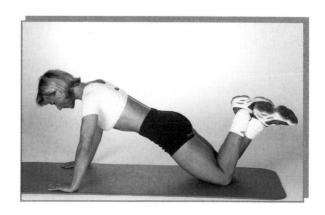

Ex.: with physiotape

Starting position:
Stepping position with your back to the wall. The physiotape is anchored below (e.g. to the wall of bars). Take both arms upwards, bending your lower arms backwards and keeping them close to your head.

Final position:
Lower arms are stretched upwards.

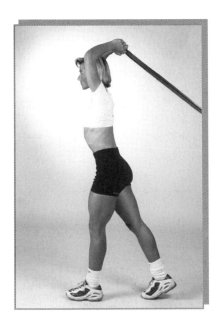

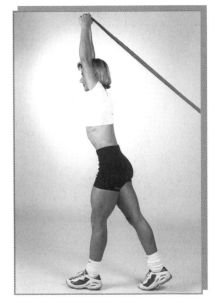

12.2 Abdominal and Back Muscles

Well-strengthened abdominal muscles can be seen as having an aesthetic as well as a healthy significance. Abdominal and back muscles constitute a human beings muscular corset, and strengthening them regularly should be a fixed component of every training session. The most important muscles are, amongst others, the straight abdominal muscle with its primary function of rolling up the body and keeping the pelvis upright, and the outer and inner abdominal muscles with their main functions: sideways bending, rotation, rolling up the body.

The back muscles also have a prime function with regard to stabilizing the spinal column every day, during sport and in general posture. The back stretcher is a collection of many small muscles which keep the individual vertebrae together, lie close to the spine and whose general functon is to keep the spine upright. The wide back muscles, the quadrilateral turning muscle and the rhomboid muscle move mainly the collar bone and the arms. The rhomboid muscles, as well as the hooded muscles help to pull the shoulder blades together backwards, and they also assist the body towards an upright position.

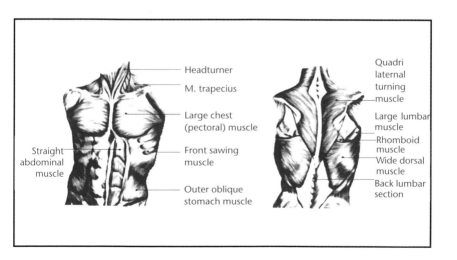

Diagram 24: Body muscles modified according to: GEIGER, SCHMID, 1997, p. 42

Ex.:

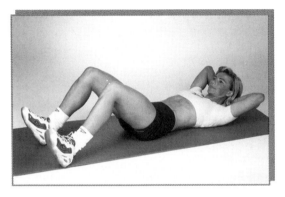

Starting position:
Lying in supine position with legs pulled up and heels pressing against the mat. Put both arms behind your neck to ease pressure on the neck muscles.

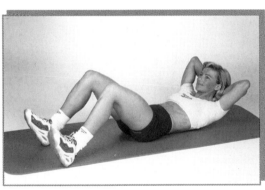

Final position 1:
Keep your body straight and lift it towards the shoulder blades. Head remains in line with your spine.

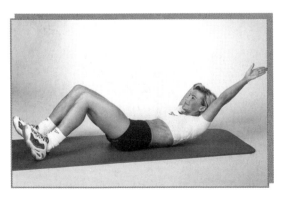

Final position 2:
See final position 1. One arm is then stretched out behind you (the more intensive version).

Ex.:

Starting position:
Lying in supine position, pull one leg towards your body and stretch out the other leg forwards and diagonally. Keep both arms behind your neck.

Final position 1:
Stretch your legs out alternately diagonally.

Final position 2:
Turn your upper body onto its side then, supporting yourself on one upper arm, stretch your legs out alternately from a slanting position.

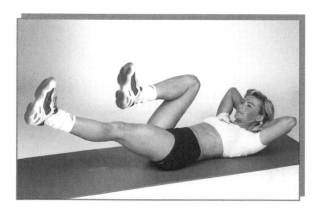

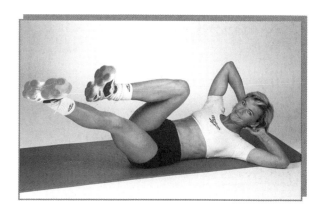

Ex.:

Starting position:
Lying in supine position with your right arm behind your neck, put your left arm on the floor with the palm of your hand pointing towards the ceiling. Pull up your right thigh and put your outside left ankle on your right thigh.

Final position:
Your right shoulder is slowly raised diagonally towards your left knee but not put down flat.

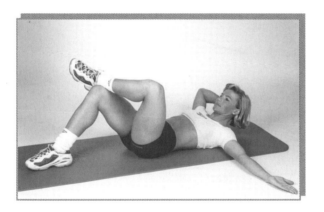

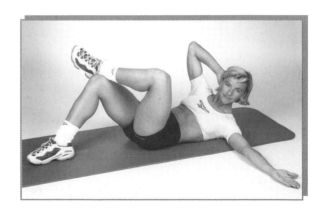

Ex.:

Starting position:
Lying in supine position, cross both legs and then lift them, bringing your thighs close to your body and keeping your arms behind your neck.

Final position:
Raise your pelvis.

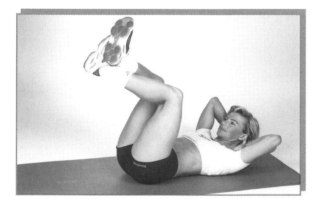

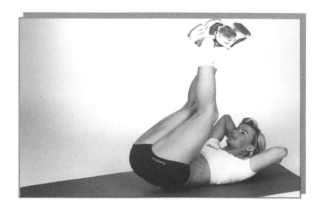

Ex.:

Starting position:
Lying in supine position, pull up your right leg and lift your bend left leg .
Put your left arm behind your neck and push your left thigh lightly with your right hand.

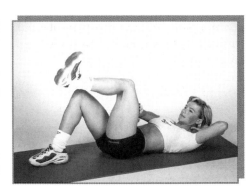

Final position:
Apply firm pressure to the left thigh with your right hand (about 10 seconds).

Ex.:with physiotape

Starting position:
In a stepping position. The physiotape is anchored at the same height as your head (e.g. at the wall bars). Stretch your arms out above your body.

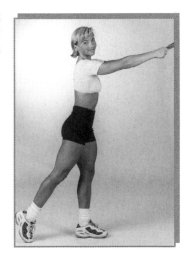

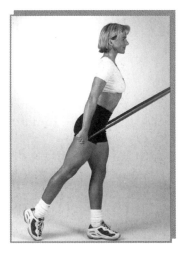

Final position:
Arms are taken down and backwards against the opposition from above and with a slight inward rotation of the shoulder joint. Wrists remain an extension of the lower arm.

Ex.: with physiotape

Starting position:
In a stepping position. The pyhsiotape is fixed at chest height (e.g. to the wall bars). Stretch out your arms forwards at shoulder height and pull the tubes taut.

Final position:
Bring your elbows backwards, and your shoulder blades at the same time slowly towards the spine, moving your sternum forwards.

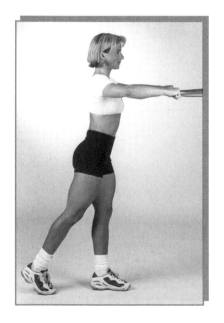

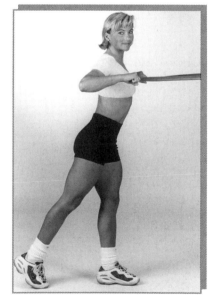

Ex.: with physiotape

Starting position:
In a stepping position with your back to the wall and the physiotape fixed to the wall bar at head level. Bend your arms and left them, pulling your elbows backwards and thus bringing your shoulder blades together.

Final position:
Both arms are stretched out forwards with the back of your hands facing the ceiling.

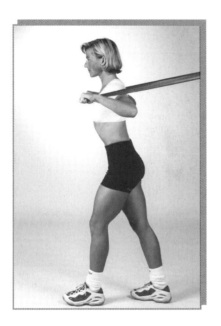

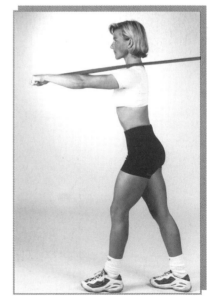

Ex.

Starting position:
Lying in prone position, put your feet on the ground in line with your hips, keeping leg, stomach and bottom muscles tense. Bend your arms into a U-shape keeping your head in line with your spine, and then pull your shoulder blades together.

Final position:
The bent arms are slowly stretched out forwards and crossed in front of your head with the back of your hands facing the ceiling.

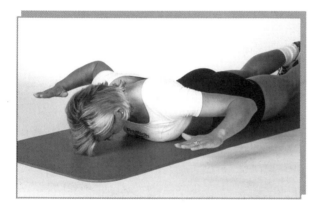

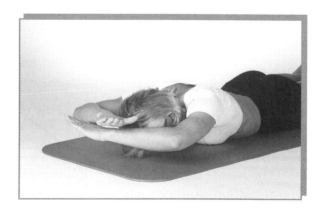

12.3 Leg and Bottom Muscles

Leg and bottom muscles which have been well-strengthened keep hip and knee joints stabilized, take some of the load off the hip joints and kneecaps, as well as keeping the pelvis physiologically in place i.e. upright.

The large bottom muscle is responsible for keeping the pelvis upright and bringing the legs into back position. The front thigh muscles are mainly responsible for stretching the knee joint and bending the hip joint.

The rear muscles main job is to bend the knee and stretch the hip. The inside of the thigh, the adductors, pull the leg back towards the body and the outside of the thigh, the abductors, lift the leg sideways.

With help from the calf muscles you can then stand on the balls of your feet.

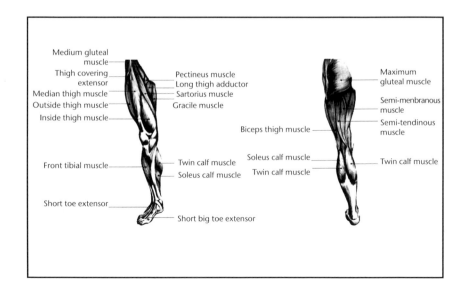

Diagram 25: Leg and bottom muscles
modified according to GEIGER, SCHMID, 1997, p. 70

Ex.: with physio tube ring

Starting position:
Lying in supine position with your legs stretched upwards, bend the knee joints slightly and draw your thighs close to your body.

Final position:
Both legs are pushed outwards.

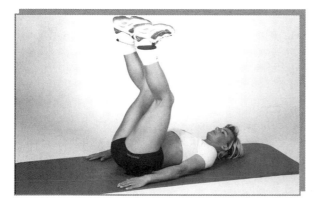

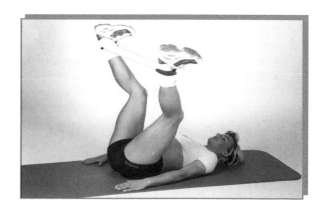

Ex.: with physio tube ring

Starting position:
Lying in supine position, bring one leg along the mat towards you. Bend the "playing" leg to an angle of 90° and raise it slightly off the mat. Pull the tip of your foot towards you.

Final position:
"Playing" leg is stretched out forwards and lifted diagonally at the same time.

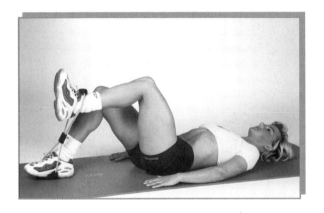

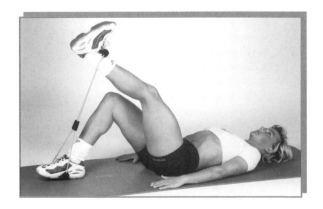

Ex.: with physio power tubes

Starting position:
Standing on one leg, bend both knee joints slightly.

Final position:
The "playing" leg is stretched out sideways.

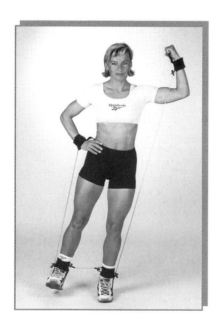

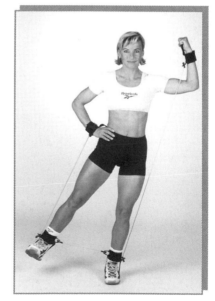

Ex.: with physio power tube

Starting position:
Standing on one leg and holding onto a chair, bend the stationary leg slightly and lift the "playing" leg bent at the knee.

Final position:
Bring the "playing" leg bent backwards and consciously tense your bottom muscles. When you lift your leg, the body is in line with itself.

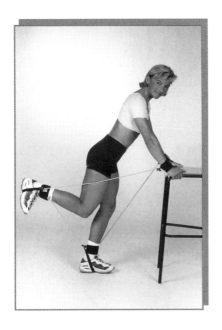

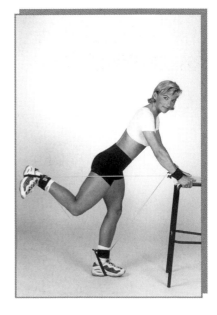

Ex.:

Starting position:
Lying in supine position, put your right leg bent on the mat and stretch your left leg upwards, keeping your arms lying beside your body.

Final position:
The left leg is stretched out towards the ceiling and your bottom lifted.

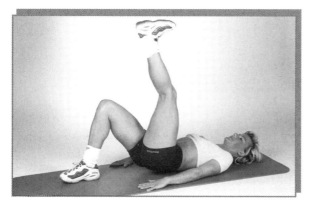

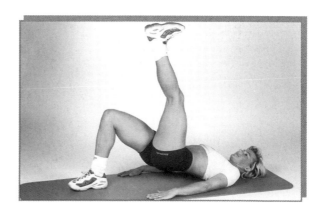

Ex.: with physio tube ring

Starting position:
Lying on your side with both legs slightly bent, draw the tips of your toes towards you. Lift your upper leg about 10 cm.

Final position:
The upper leg is lifted slowly against resistance from the physio tube ring.

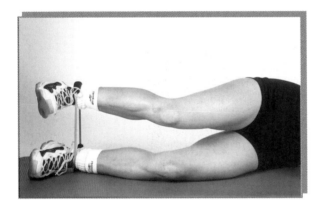

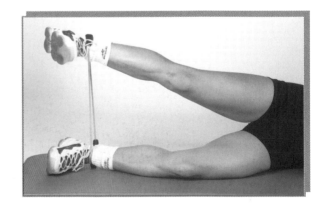

Ex.:

Starting position:
Lying on your side, bend your upper leg and put it down in front of you on a raised surface (e.g. a ball, step etc). Stretch out your lower leg in line with your body. Stretch out your lower arm flat along the floor and put your head on that upper arm.

Final position:
Lift your lower leg, whilst still stretched out, off the floor and then lower it again but do not put it right down.

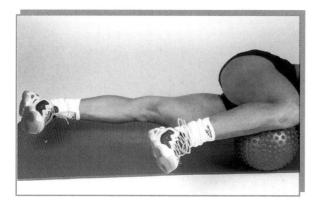

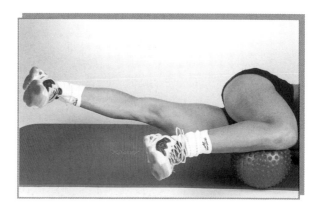

Ex.:

Starting position:
Quadruped press-ups supported on your lower arms with both elbows below the shoulder joints. Raise one leg with it bent.

Final position:
The "playing" leg is first stretched out backwards and then raised until making one line with your body. Your head remains an extension of your spine.

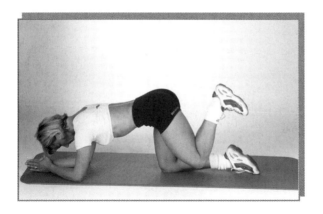

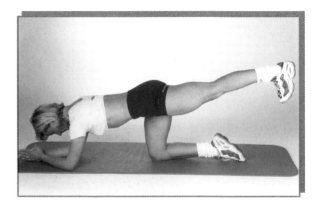

Ex.:

Starting position:
Quadruped press-ups supported on your lower arms with both elbows below the shoulder joints. Bend one leg and lift it into a horizontal position.

Final position:
Move the diagonally bent leg downwards (onto the other side).

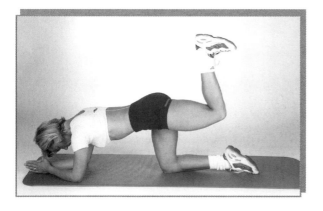

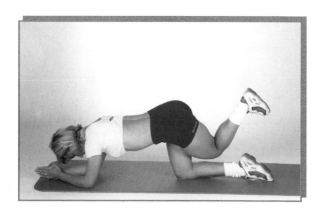

Ex.:

Starting position:
Lying in supine position with both legs pulled up the mat towards you and arms lying beside you on the ground, raise your pelvis.

Final position:
The pelvis is raised slightly until it is in line with your body. Consciously tense your bottom muscles whilst lifting.

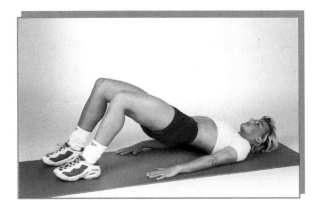

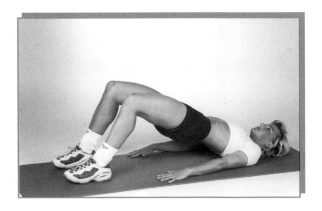

13 Stretching

Make stretching a definite part of your warming-up and cooling-down programme and use muscle stretching to relax. If you stretch properly, you will not overtax or injure yourself. The stretching position should last between 20 and 60 seconds. Repeat each exercise at best twice. You should stretch the groups of muscles which you have been strengthening most intensively, as well as the muscles especially inclined to become shorter (see chapter 6.3).

Arm and shoulder muscles

Ex.:

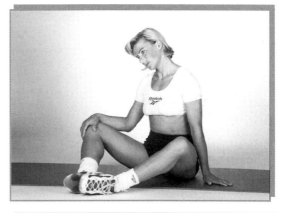

Sitting upright, with your heels close to your body, bring the soles of your feet together. Let your knees fall loosely to the sides. Tilt your head sideways, whilst actively pulling your other shoulder downwards.
This can be varied with other chin positions. Sense the stretching in the muscles at the side of your neck and at the back of your neck.

Ex.:

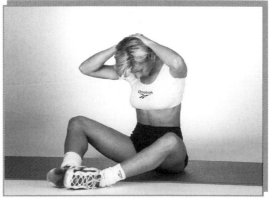

Sitting upright, tilt your head forwards and support your hands by moving carefully. Sense the stretching at the back of your neck and in your upper back.

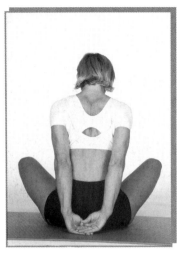

Ex.:

Sitting upright with your arms behind your back, pull them up your back with palms facing upwards. Vary the position of your arms e.g. bring them up at your side diagonally.
Feel the stretching in your chest muscles and the tension in your back muscles.

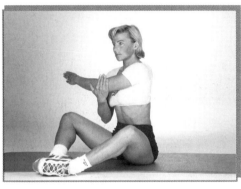

Ex.:

Sitting upright, pull your arm stretched out towards your body and increase the stretching with your other hand. The inner rotators of the shoulder joint are then stretched. Variation: Twist your arm, so that your little finger is pointing upwards; then the outer rotators of the shoulder joint are stretched.

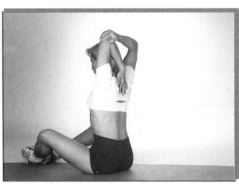

Ex.:

Sitting upright, one arm is bent and taken over your head towards your shoulder blade. The other hand then clasps your elbow, pulling it down towards the back of your head. Your rear upper arm is being stretched.

Trunk muscles

Ex.:

Knee stand. Open your knees inline with your pelvis and tilt your upper body forward in a relaxed way to look between your legs. By moving your hands you can intensify the stretching. Sense the stretching in your back.

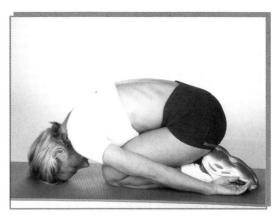

Ex.:

Lying in supine position with arms and legs stretched out as far as possible, make yourself as long as possible. Maintain physiological lordosis.
Sense the stretching in your stomach.

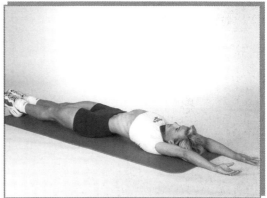

Variation:

Move your upper body and legs sideways (slight arched tension). Both shoulders and heels remain in contact with the floor. Feel the stretching in your sides.

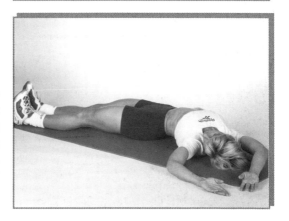

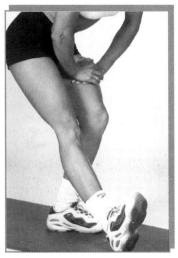

Leg and bottom muscles

Ex.:

Whilst standing, put your pelvis at a 90° angle to your outstretched leg. Tilt your pelvis forwards and keep your back straight. Stretch one leg out forwards, pulling the tip of your foot towards you, and supporting your weight on the other thigh, so as not to overload your back. Feel the stretching in your rear thigh.

or Ex.:

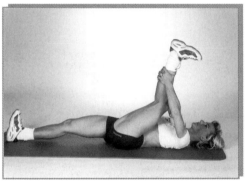

Lying in supine position with one leg stretched out on the floor and the other leg stretched upwards, pull this leg towards your body with both arms but not at the knee joint. To intensify the exercise, pull the tip of your foot towards you and in-crease the leg stretching.

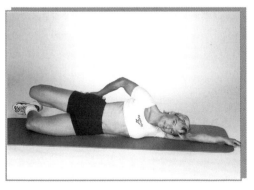

Ex.:

Lying on your side. Bend your lower leg putting it behind you. Pull you upper lower leg towards your bottom, pushing your pelvis forwards. Feel the stretching in your hip and front of your thigh.

Ex.:

Huge lunge forward. Bring your upper body onto your thigh, with one hand for support on the floor. Press your hip towards the floor, letting your body weight fall forwards so that pressure on the rear of your knee is minimal. Push your rear leg back as far as possible. Feel the stretching in your side hip muscle.

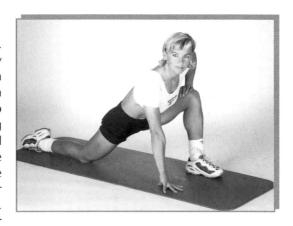

Ex.:

Lying in supine position, stretch both legs out sideways and then intensify this by applying slight pressure outwards with both arms. Feel the stretching on the inside of your thighs.

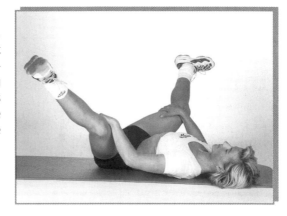

14 Remarks to the Apparatus Used

Training with additional apparatus leads to an improvement in one's general physical capacity. All basic motoric characteristics like endurance, strength, speed, co-ordination and mobility can be effectively increased. Especially in the area of strength development, one can move out effectively from a higher level of training. One big advantage with the physioline is that young and old, weak and strong performers, newcomers and the advanced, can all use these apparatus, because they have varying degrees of pull to choose from. The following manual apparatus are amongst the most modern training devices in the whole fitness area.

1 Physio Power Tube (PPT):
PPT is a universal aerobic and workout device with a high level of effectiveness for one's fitness and strength-building. It consists of a leg-tube which is fixed to both ankles with a velcro strip, as well as the two arm-tubes, fitted to wrist cuffs and joined up again to leg cuffs.

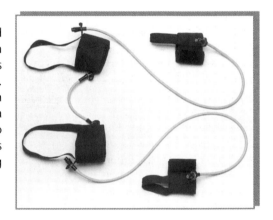

2 Physio Tube Toner:
The physio tube toner is a versatile piece of hand apparatus to intensify by special training of individual groups of muscles. The toner is compact and easy to hold, has various uses and can be stored easily, making it an ideal training device for home, in a fitness studio or on a journey.

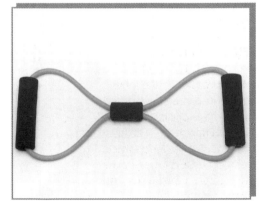

3 Physio Tube Basic:

A physio tube is a strength pulling device belonging to the most modern pieces of equipment in the fitness area. An increase in one's general performance potential by training all the big and important muscle groups is enhanced by an improvement in one's co-ordinative ability.

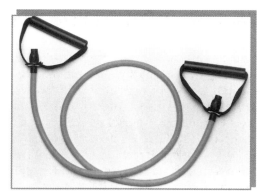

4 Physioband:

The physioband is a progressive latex band for therapy and fitness, which is useful as an open as well as a closed system with a patented fixing clip. The physiobands come in five different strengths for resistance exercises which can be built up one after the other as required. It is ideally suited to improving one's general fitness, for more strength, endurance and better co-ordination.

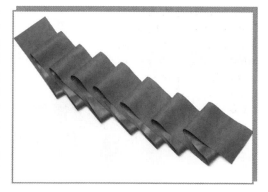

5 Physio Tube Ring:

The physio tube ring is a further product in the physio range and consists of a closed system made of latex with two soft foam handles. It is possible by using this hand-held device, to train muscle groups in the context of continually improved performance.

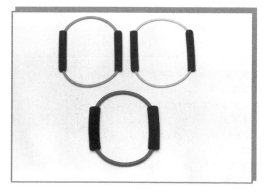

6 Physio Bar:

The physio bar is a general training device for strengthening the muscles. The physio bar consists of an adjustable latex tube, a movable bar and belongs to the group of modern apparatus, which can be easily used at home, on journeys and in a fitness studio.

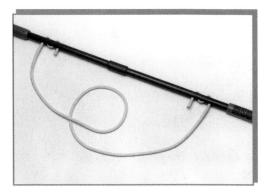

15 Epilogue

Establish the goals you wish to attain in both your home and working life. Check whether goals like visiting friends, finishing a computer course or sticking photos into an album can be realized within a given space of time. If you have managed to complete this plan successfully, then set yourself new goals, which you can systematically work towards, including for example the fitness programme. Regard it as an important part of the route to visibly improving your health, your figure and general well-being, because without your health you will achieve very few of your aims in life.

The combined effect of specific training, healthy eating and ant-cellulite care is the best tip I can give for having smooth legs and a firm bottom. You now have all the knowledge at your disposal of what to do to treat cellulite. Now it is up to you alone to change your attitude towards health and fitness. Don't let your life be ruled by unwanted bulges of fat; get on and do something about it, then your level of well-being and optimism will increase.

"New realms can come into being, when old habits change"
Tuli KUPFERBERG

By the way: Legs need movement – that's what they're made for!

I wish you every success in your future efforts.

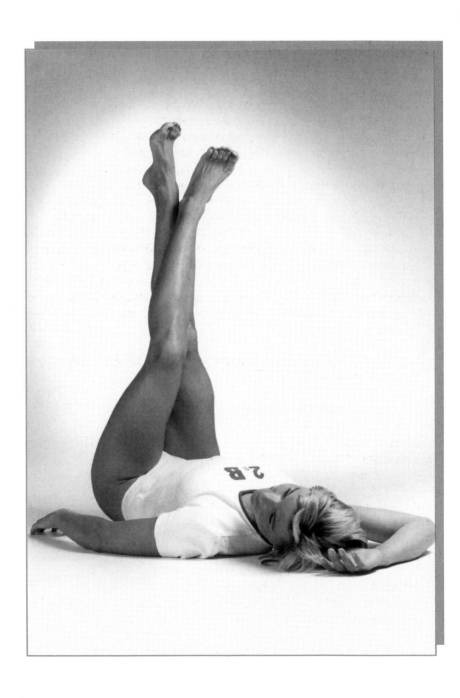

16 Bibliography

1. BAILEY, C.: Fett verlieren – Form gewinnen. Meyer & Meyer 1996.

2. BERNSTEIN, D./BORKOVEC, T.: Entspannungstraining – Handbuch der progressiven Muskelentspannung. München 1987.

3. BRENNER, H.: Entspannungs-Training. Humboldt 1982.

4. BURKE, K.: Schmale Hüften – Schlanke Beine. Mosaik-Verlag 1995.

5. BUSKIES, W./BOECKH-BEHRENS, W.: Gesundheitsorientiertes Fitnesstraining Band 1,2,3. Dr. Loges + Co Winsen 1996.

6. DENOTH, J./STACOFF, A.: Belastung und Beanspruchung der Muskulatur. In: Sportverl.-Sportschad./5 (1991), Georg Thieme Verlag Stuttgart. New York, 17-21.

7. FALLER, A.: Der Körper des Menschen – Einführung in Bau und Funktion. Stuttgart 1995.

8. „Fit und schön im Sommer". In: Brigitte Zeitschrift, 10/98, S. 52.

9. FRESE, H./GUTSCHENREITER, I.: Das große Handbuch der vegetarischen Vollwert-Ernährung. Itzehoe 1993.

10. FÜRST, I.: Wettlauf um den Markt der Fettleibigkeit. In: Deutsches Ärzteblatt 93, Heft 12, 22. März 1996.

11. GEIGER, U./SCHMID, C.: Muskeltraining mit dem Thera-Band, BLV aktiv & gesund, 1997.

12. HAUNER, H.: Gesundheitsrisiken von Übergewicht und Gewichtszunahme. In: Deutsches Ärzteblatt 93, Heft 51-52, 23, Dezember 1996.

13. „Haut und Figur". In: Sonderheft, Journal für die Frau, 2/98.

14. HELLMIß, M.: Das große Praxisbuch – Apfelessig. Südwest Verlag 1997.

15. HOTTENROTT, K.: Ausdauertraining. Dr. Loges + Co, Winsen 1995.

16. HUETHER, G./SCHMIDT, S./RÜTHER, E.: Essen, Serotonin und Psyche. In: Deutsches Ärzteblatt 95, Heft 9,27. Februar 1998.

17. HUSEMANN, B.: Die chirurgische Therapie der extremen Adipositas. In: Deutsches Ärzteblatt 94, Heft 33, 15. August 1997.

18. KOCH, CH.: „Iss dich glücklich, rauch dich froh". In: Stern 26/98, S. 107.

19. KITAJEW-SMYK, L.: Psychologia stresu. Wydawnictwo, Wroclaw 1989.

20. KRAFT, W./ SCHOBER, H./ SCHMIDT, H./ WITTEKOPF, G.: Stretching und muskuläres Entspannungsverhalten am Muskulus quadratus femoris. In: Zeitschrift für Physiotherapie 42 (1990), 237-243.

21. KREMPEL, O.: Anti Cellulite Training. Rowohlt, Hamburg 1994.

22. KREMPEL, O.: Bodytrainer für die Frau ab 50. Rowohlt, Hamburg 1997.

23. MARKERT, D.: Die Markert Diät, endlich Schluß mit dem Jo-Jo-Effekt. Goldmann, 1996.

24. MÜLLER, E.: Entspannungsmethoden in der Rehabilitation. Erlangen 1987.

25. OBERBEIL, K/LENTZ, C.: Obst und Gemüse als Medizin. Südwest, 1997.

26. PAUL, G./SCHUBA, V.: Aktiv kontra Osteoporose. Meyer & Meyer 1998.

27. Pschyrembel – Klinisches Wörterbuch. de Gruyter 1986.

28. RONSARD, N.: Das Anti-Cellulite-Erfolgsprogramm. Rowohlt 1997.

29. RÜDIGER, M./HÄBERLEIN, S: Problemzonen. Falken 1996.

30: „Schlank für immer". In: Fit for Fun, 10/97, S. 24.

31. Schröder, E.M.: Wasser: Lebenselixier – nicht nur für Sportler. In: Krankengymnastik (KG) 49, Nr. 8, 1997.

32. Schröder, E.M.: Vitamine. In: Krankengymnastik (KG) 49, Nr. 1, 1997.

33. Spitzweg, C. u.a.: Physiologische und pathophysiologische Bedeutung von Leptin beim Menschen. In: Deutsches Ärzteblatt 94, Heft 44, 31. Oktober 1997.

34. Wechsler, J.-G. u.a.: Therapie der Adipositas. In: Deutsches Ärzteblatt 93, Heft 36,6. September 1996.

35. Wechsler, J.-G.: Diätetische Therapie der Adipositas. In: Deutsches Ärzteblatt 94, Heft 36,5. September 1997.

36. Wiemann, K.: Stretching, Grundlagen, Möglichkeiten, Grenzen. In: Sportunterricht, Schorndorf, 42 (1993), Heft 3, 91-106.

17 Glossary

adipocytes – fatty cell tissues which are genetically fixed. In fat addicts, individual cells have more fat in them.

adipose - fatty, have a high fat content

adiposity - obesity; state of being too fat

aerobic – with oxygen delivery

anaerobic – without oxygen delivery

androgen – steroid hormone and a collective term for male sex hormones e.g. testerone.

anorexia – loss of appetite, lowering of the usual drive to eat; can occur during mouth-, stomach-, gut- and infectious diseases and in pregnancy.

anorexia nervosa – an addiction to being thin in puberty; a psychogenic eating disorder with a distorted view of food intake, food and one's weight, a disturbed outlook on one's body, fear of overweight and denying being ill.

antagonists – muscles which work contra to the acting synergists and put a brake on our movements.

basic turnover – the production of energy necessary to maintain organ function. This is independent of age, sex, surface of the body, hormonal function or type of diet.
Can be increased by fever, tumours, pregnancy, overactive thyroid gland, hunger etc.

bulimia – being ravenously hungry, eating addiction.

bulimia nervosa – addiction to eating and then being sick; a psychogenic eating disorder where excessive amounts of highly calorific food are consumed in a very short time, and after which measures are taken to try and keep the body weight within its normal limits (e.g. alternating with periodic fasting or following the eating binges with self-induced being sick or the misuse of laxatives or diuretics).

cardiovascular – concerned with the heard and blood vessels.

chromosomes – little inherited particles visibly carrying inherited features. The genes are arranged in lines on the chromosomes (dictating our hereditary features). Each human being has 23 pairs of chromosomes.

collagen – "scaffolding" protein which appears for example in the connective tissue, tendons, ligaments, cartilage and bones.

contraction – pulling together e.g. of a muscle.

cutis – skin

distress – negative stress which makes us ill.

elastin – protein "scaffolding" material

electrolytes – compounds (acids, base products, satls) which accelerate chemical reactions.

enzymes –proteins which appear as catalytic converters in living organisms and which accelerate chemical reactions. Orderly metabolism and therefore life in general would be impossible without enzymes.

epidermis – the outermost layer of skin

epithel tissue – a closed single or layered band of cells, which covers inner or outer surfaces of the body. Functions: protection, metabolic exchange, reception of stimuli.

eustress – good, positive, vital stress

extra-cellular – outside the cell

gestagen – a hormone which works together with oestrogen to regulate the reproductive processes of the female genital organs.

hormones – information carriers for the various types of cells within the organism.

One can differentiate between two main groups:
1. steroid hormones e.g. oestrogen, testosterone, progesterone, glucocorticoide, aldosterone etc. and
2. polypeptide hormones like oxytocin, insulin, parathormone, calzitonin and two sibsidiary groups: the amines (adrenalin, noradrenalin, thyroxin, acetylcholin) and the unsaturated fatty acids (prostaglandine).

hyaluron acid – is an inter-cellular type of putty important as a basic substance in the connective tussue.

hypertrophie – enlargement of individual cells and sections of tissue without any significant increase in size (e.g. muscular hypertropie).

immobilisation – putting at rest/ out of action

intermittent – in short bursts with pauses.

intermuscular co-ordination – interplay of motor units of various muscles.

interstitial – situated between the tissues.

interstitium – an intermediate space containing connective tissue, blood vessels and nerves.

intracellular – within the cell

intramuscular co-ordination – interplay between the muscle cells of various motor units in any one muscle.

lactate – salt of milk acid; normal venous amount up to 1.3 mmol/l, i.e. about 12 mg/100 ml.

leptin – hormone to make one feel full.

leptose – thin

lipides – fats

lipoedema – symmetrical painful oedema found especially in women's hips.

lipos – Greek for fat

lymphatic drainage – a type of massage by stroking to get rid of lymphatic blockages; one strokes the skin with one's finger-tips along the lymph vessels.

lymphatic fluid – a pale yellow fluid consisting of lymph plasma and lymph corpuscels, which more or less correspond with the lymphocytes. Lymphatic fluid is made by blood plasma leaving th blood capillaries and coming into the tissue. The amount is independent of the extent of the pressure in the blood capillaries and can be increased by the activity of any organ especially the muscles. It then flows into gaps in the tissues and is taken back into the blood stream by special vessels (the lymphatic vessels) via the local lymph nodes.

lymphocytes – the smallest white blood corpuscles, acting as immunity carriers, and thus of vital importance for the body's immunity system; about 70% of them are to be found in the lymphatic organs (lymph nodes, spleen, thymus gland and tonsils), 10% in the bone marrow, 4% in the blood and 10-20% in other tissues.

melancytes – cells capable of forming melanin in the basal layer of the epidermis.

melanin – dark pigments containing nitrogen, which caused by oxidation and determine skin and hair colour and the colour of the iris in the eye.

metabolic – stemming from metabolism

minute ventilation – the volume of air which can be breathed in or out during 1 minute peaceful breathing. Calculation: frequency per minute x volume of breath; normal amount about 8 litres.

obese – high fat content

obesity – the state of being too fat

oedema – water retention, painless and non-inflammatory swellings as a result of watery fluid collecting in the gaps between the tissues e.g. in the skin and mucous membranes.

oestrogen – steroid hormones which are formed in the ovaries, follicles, in the placenta and in the testicides. The most important physiological oestrogens are oestradiol, oestron and oestriol.
All the female reproductive processes are regulated by oestrogen and gestagen (e.g. maturing of the follicles, egg transport, making the walls of the vagina etc) and they also stimulate the bone maturation process, check the function of the sebaceous glands and cause water retention.

osteoporosis – a quantitative reduction of the bone tissue also known as bone atrophy.

progesterone – a steroid hormone (gestagen hormone) which, in combination with oestrogen, can cause an egg cell to ripen and be transported.

retentio – holding back

synergists – muscles which do the same job.

18 Subject Index

Health & Fitness!

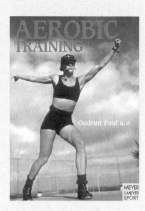

Gudrun Paul a.o.
Aerobic Training

This book deals with the general principals of fitness training, as well as those specifically belonging to aerobics.

The reader can see how to build up a series of lessons in aerobics training with many practical examples and, in particular, various basic steps and their technical application are introduced.

At the same time, ways of communication – method and cueing – are described and the book also shows many ways of varying aerobics training.

160 pages
126 photos, 16 figures
paperback, 14.8 x 21 cm
ISBN 1-84126-021-5
£ 12.95 UK/$ 17.95 US/
$ 25.95 CDN

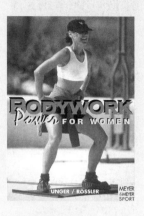

Edgar Unger/Jürgen Rössler
Bodywork – Power for Women

This book provides a comprehensive programme and detailed work-out instructions so that you can change your figure according to the goals you set yourself, stay younger in a biological way – and healthier. It also helps to arrest a decline in sporting activity and suggests how to improve fitness through a variety of exercises and training programmes in the illustrated training section.

Finally, the book provides a variety of helpful tips for women on equipment, nutrition and motivation.

144 pages
76 figures
paperback, 14.8 x 21 cm
ISBN 1-84126-022-3
£ 12.95 UK/$ 17.95 US/
$ 25.95 CDN

MEYER
MEYER
SPORT

MEYER & MEYER Verlag | Von-Coels-Straße 390 | D-52080 Aachen, Germany | Fax ++49(0)241/9 58 10 1

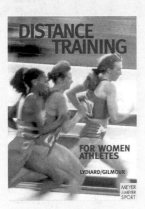

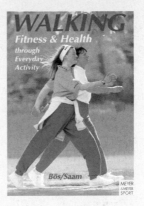

Arthur Lydiard/Garth Gilmour
Distance Training for Women Athletes

This book provides a comprehensive explanation of the principles of training, both physiological and mechanical, clothing, equipment and diet, and the avoidance of, and treatment for, injuries. Changes to the body which specifically affect women are discussed and the book also contains details of the difference and the balance between aerobic and anaerobic training and the use of training variations, such as fartlek, hill training, resistance training and speed work.

128 pages, 43 photos
14.8 x 21 cm
ISBN 1-84126-002-9
£ 9.95 UK/$ 14.95 US/
$ 20.95 CDN

Klaus Bös/Joachim Saam
Walking
Fitness & Health through Everyday Activity

Walking is introduced as an especially health-promoting kind of sport, which anyone can indulge in. This book describes the basics of walking technique, considers the necessary clothing, the appropriate medical background, and also gives advice on diet.
It provides interesting incentives for the professional as well as the beginner, like schemes for strengthening the whole body or tips for new kinds of walking e.g. body walking (meditative walking).

112 pages, 20 photos
paperback, 11.5 x 18 cm
ISBN 1-84126-001-0
£ 5.95 UK/$ 8.95 US/
$ 12.95 CDN

If you are interested in **Meyer & Meyer Sport** and its large programme, please visit us **online** or call our **Hotline** and order our catalogue!

online:
▶ www.meyer-meyer-sports.com

Hotline:
▶ + + 49 (0)1 80/5 10 11 15

We are looking forward to your call!

MEYER
& MEYER
SPORT

MEYER & MEYER Verlag | Von Coels Straße 390 | D-52080 Aachen, Germany | Fax + +49 (0)241/9 58 10 10